Trave... he...

A travel health guide
for the general practitioner
and the travel clinic nurse

Travel, trauma, risks and health promotion:

A travel health guide
for the general practitioner
and the travel clinic nurse

by
Iain B McIntosh

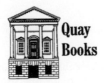

Quay
Books

Quay Books Division, Mark Allen Publishing Group
Jesses Farm, Snow Hill, Dinton, Wiltshire, SP3 5HN

British Library Cataloguing-in-Publication Data
A catalogue record is available for this book

© Mark Allen Publishing Ltd 1998
ISBN 1 85642 085 X

Printed in the UK by Redwood Books, Trowbridge, Wiltshire.

Contents

Acknowledgements

I wish to thank my wife and Pamela my daughter for their tolerance and support in the writing of this book.

Permission to use material from some of my published articles in Travel Medicine International for some of these chapters is gratefully acknowledged.

Preface

There is more to travel medicine than malaria.

(L'Etang, 1995)

A cursory appraisal of the literature might not support the above assertion. Articles on malaria and vaccine-preventable disease swamp the journals and generate much controversy. Although important, these diseases account for a fraction of the morbidity and mortality in people travelling abroad.

Vaccine-preventable disease is responsible for only five percent of travel-related illness. Travellers are far more likely to suffer from diarrhoea and accidental trauma. Simple precautions can minimise many of the increased health risks to which overseas travellers are liable. Although diarrhoea and accidents are common, certain groups of travellers are at higher risk.

The backpacker, adventurer, camper, explorer and climber are all more susceptible. So, too, are those who practice their sport on beaches, seas, rivers and high mountains in exotic and remote places. These travellers face increased risk of exposure to physical, physiological and psychological travel-related health hazards.

In pre-travel health consultations, more than advice on malaria or appropriate immunisations should be given. The needs of travellers should be identified and targeted. The health professional's consultation should offer advice and support, specific to these needs. This book considers these higher risk travellers, the health hazards to which they may be exposed and appropriate precautionary advice to ensure that they return home in good health.

Introduction

The primary objectives of travel medicine are:

▶ to keep travellers alive and healthy

▶ to minimise the impact of overseas illness and accidents.

These goals should be achieved by:

▼ pre-travel preparations

▼ prophylaxis

▼ behaviour modification

▼ self-treatment and care.

Mainstays of the discipline depend on:

● information sharing and education — primarily on food, water, flies and other insects, infections and potential trauma

● immunisations

● chemoprophylaxis

● therapy for contracted illness.

Travel medicine is a new discipline which is very much a product of this decade. It is fuelled by the increasing numbers travelling world-wide on business or leisure, increasing affluence, longer retirement, larger, faster aeroplanes and bigger and more luxurious cruise liners. In the millenium the 750-seat aeroplane and the 4000-passenger cruise ship will be in service.

Tourists are extending the range of their holidays from short-haul continental travel to more exotic and remote destinations. The hygiene standards and health facilities which are common in the United Kingdom are less common in much of the developing world. There sanitation is often elementary and hygiene is governed by the availability of water. Public safety is a minor concern and medical facilities and emergency services may be embryonic. Most holiday-makers are oblivious to these risks until an accident or illness occurs and they are then faced with the reality of scarce or absent resources.

Good travel medicine practice is of most import for those visiting areas, such as developing, tropical and semitropical countries, high altitudes, and places where extremes of heat, humidity or freezing temperatures, found in deserts, jungles or sub-Arctic conditions are common. In the past, such destinations were the prerogative of scientists or the privilege of the wealthy. With the availability of cheap travel, these regions are now included in the itineraries of trekking, climbing, adventure and exploring groups . The very young, the teenager, the middle-aged and the very old visit some of the remotest parts of the world.

Recently, when exploring a disused British Antarctic survey post, I met a group which included a 1-year-old child and an 88-year-old woman, who were visiting the ice-cap. Extreme cold seems no longer a barrier to global exploration.

Approximately 35 million people from industrialised countries visit the developing world annually (Steffen and Dupont, 1994). Eighty percent are tourists and many are remarkably ignorant of the substructure and service facilities of the country they are visiting. Some are concerned about their health when away from home, fearing gastric or other food/water borne disorders. They take prophylactics and treat their symptoms promptly. Others exhibit fears and travel-related anxieties which may be psychological but can still be of major concern (McIntosh *et al*, 1996) see *Chapter 9.*

The effects of travel on the individual

Travellers often fail to appreciate where the real risks to their health lie. More tourists will suffer from vehicle and pedestrian accidents or sports-induced trauma than from travel-induced infections. Few appreciate the inadequacy of the medical resources available, particularly in developing countries. The importance of the role of the travel health professional to educate and advise on the risks and means of minimising these cannot be overstated.

The more adventurous may suffer physical trauma, physiological disturbance from travel sickness, fluid loss, dehydration and upset to circadian rhythms on their journeys. A large number of travellers report psychological upset and travel-related anxieties when abroad or en route. These problems and some of the means which the travel health counsellor can employ to diminish them, are considered in this book.

Regular business travellers do not necessarily escape from the risks of travel. The traditional focus on the effects of business pressures may not be completely justified. International travel can pose health risks beyond exposure to infectious diseases. It has been noted that business travellers file medical claims more frequently than non-business travellers, and this applies to many categories of disease and trauma. The number of claims increase with the frequency of travel. Trauma is a common feature, and back injury claims are higher in male travellers, possibly due to carrying heavy luggage and sitting in aircraft for prolonged periods (Liese *et al*, 1997).

Claims due to psychological diagnoses are three times higher in male travellers and twice as high in women travellers who have completed two business trips. Some long-distance travellers suffer from stress caused by the sudden changes in climate, daily activities, food, drink and sleep patterns.

Appropriate immunisations are important. The emphasis on these financially rewarding procedures has driven the upsurge in travel health clinics, but more attention should now be given to the common features which affect travellers. There is a clear need for additional research on factors, such as psychological and psychosocial responses, health practices and time-zone crossings.

Table: Introduction.1: The effects of travel on the individual

Risks	Effects
High temperature risk	*hyperthermia* *heat* *dehydration*
Low temperature risk	*hypothermia* *exposure*
Humidity	*disturbance in temperature control*
Altitude	*increased risk of acute mountain sickness* *hypoxia*
Disturbances in circadian rhythm	*mental change* *disturbed metabolism*
Air travel	*low partial pressure of oxygen* *dry air* *contaminated air*
Sea/land/air transport-ation	*motion sickness*
Cultural shock	*psychological distress*
Environmental stress	*noise, delay, re-routing and baggage loss can cause confusion and mental distress*

Risks	Effects
Communication problems	*linguistic and public address systems can cause misunderstanding and subsequent mental distress*
Travel fatigue	*modern air travel can cause fatigue and psychological disturbance*
Physical stress	*long airport walkways, carrying suitcases, climbing stairs are all physically demanding*
Enforced immobility	*can cause venous thrombosis and pulmonary embolism*
Risk of disease	*tropical illnesses which are controlled in the United Kingdom can be contracted in under-developed countries*

The practice of travel medicine has been stimulated by courses, similar to that established at Glasgow University which now awards a Diploma and an MSc in Travel Medicine. Hopefully, graduates will initiate research which will answer some of the questions currently raised in the field of travel medicine. The recently established British Travel Health Association encourages all travel health professionals, travel companies and agencies to work together to improve the health and safety of people travelling overseas by founding an educational source for doctors and nurses who are active in this field. Health care professionals have a responsibility to counsel and educate travellers so that they may return home in good health.

References

L'Etang H (1995) Editorial. *Trav Med Int* **13**: 4

Liese B, Mundt A, Dell L, *et al* (1997) Medical insurance claims associated with international business travel. *Occup Environ Med* **54**: 499–503

McIntosh I, Power K, Swanson V (1996) Prevalence intensity and sex differences in travel related stressors. *J Trav Med* **3**: 96–102

Steffen R, DuPont H (1994) Travel medicine. What's that? *J Trav Med* **1**: 1–3

Setting up a general practice health clinic

The number of UK travellers to remote destinations has increased by a factor of six in the last 30 years, and has caused a boom in the demand for pre-travel health advice. This increase in international travel and the subsequent growth of travel-related illness, has led to an expansion in the provision of travel health services. Many general practices have set up pre-travel health promotion clinics which offer counselling, clinical assessment, identification of medical risk, prophylaxis, vaccinations and advice tailored to the individual and his/her destination. Practice nurses often manage these clinics and play a central role in their development (McIntosh, 1995). Travel-induced illness and its prevention covers:

- vaccination and prophylaxis
- phobia-counselling
- acute mountain sickness
- jet-lag
- travel sickness and travellers diarrhoea
- trauma.

A well-run travel health clinic depends on:

- good organisation
- a sound database
- enthusiastic, skilled and experienced nurses and doctors
- careful audit.

Most UK residents travel the world in safety, but at least a third suffer from travel-induced illness and some will return home unwell. Treatment uses up valuable resources so counselling, adequate vaccination and prophylaxis can reduce the incidence of illness abroad and save on costs to the National Health Service and individual practices.

The discipline of travel medicine has evolved in response to the health needs of tourists and is a unique medical specialty (Dupont and

Steffen, 1997). The role for the primary care team in preparing people for international travel has been clearly identified as:

● preparation, precaution and protection against known potential health problems

● maintaining good health during travel

● post-travel identification and treatment of travel-induced disease.

Healthier travel

The key to healthier travel, and to decreasing the impact of travel-related illness in returning travellers, is the recognition of individual risk. Advice should be tailored to the individual, his/her destination, transport mode and lifestyle. Special efforts should be made to identify high-risk travellers.

High risk travellers

► those aged between 20 and 30 years of age who drink heavily

► those with previous and current ill-health

► pregnant women

► the elderly and very young

► backpackers and expeditioners

► high altitude climbers

► those with chronic illness and on medications

► sportsmen and women travellers.

A well-run travel clinic has clinical advantage for its users. Services, such as immunisation prophylaxis and other protective measures can be financially rewarding for general practice clinic practitioners. The following can also be offered to the traveller:

▼ first-aid kits and water purifiers

▼ AIDS protection kits, insect repellants

▼ sunscreen, mosquito nets

▼ vaccination certificates, fitness to travel certificates

▼ private travel prescriptions.

Travel-related illness may ruin the individual holiday or upset a business trip but it can also add to the management burden of primary clinical care.

Many travellers return from Africa or Asia to consult their Gps because they are still suffering from an illness (usually gastrointestinal or respiratory) which they contracted during their holiday (McIntosh *et al*, 1993). They can be treated by the staff of the travel health clinic, thus avoiding disrupting routine surgery consultations (Tilley, 1997). To run an effective travel health clinic, practice nurses, practice managers, receptionists, doctors and health visitors should all be involved.

Objectives

What objectives need to be considered before setting up a travel health clinic? These should be to:

- ▶ provide comprehensive advice on how to maintain good health
- ▶ inform travellers of possible risks
- ▶ provide immunisation and prophylaxis
- ▶ audit the post-travel presentation of illness.

Responsibilities and facilities which should be considered are listed in Table 1.1.

Table 1.1: Travel health clinics: facilities and responsibilities

staff responsibility for the different elements in the programme:

time commitment, ie. the length of each session and the number of appointments

provision of appropriate equipment, such as refrigerators

acquisition and storage of vaccines

fees for vaccinations and prophylaxis

provision of information leaflets

identification of specific travel health risks

establishment of protocols for staff, ie. assessment protocols for nurses

---

Table 1.1: Travel health clinics: facilities and responsibilities

provision of back-up support by general practitioners

education and training of staff, especially nurses, to agreed standards

criteria for acquisition of yellow fever immunisation centre status

promoting and advertising the clinic

audit of the clinic when established

Initial consultations should be allocated a 20 minute appointment. In a practice of 2000 patients, two to four hours a week should be allowed during the main holiday season, although less time can be allocated out of season. The practice can assess the demand for the clinic by conducting a sample survey of practice patients before setting up the main programme. Doctors should be available to give advice and conduct examinations where necessary.

Protocols

Organisational protocols need to be established. These will clarify the responsibilities of each member of staff, the immunisations that are to be given, and by whom, the use of patient consent forms, acquisition and storage of drugs and claims for approved immunisation. These protocols must be agreed and signed by nurses and doctors, and should authorise the nurse to perform specified tasks. In-house training will educate receptionists to direct potential travellers to the travel clinic. Receptionists and administrative secretaries will also require training on how to complete and submit claim forms to the FHSAs/Health Boards.

Well-trained nurses and clearly established protocols means that a clinic can be managed with occasional support and consultation from the doctor. Destinations and travel data should be assessed so that specific programmes of immunisations and travel advice management protocols can be set up. Provision of general and specific advice will be the nurse's responsibility.

The doctor's role

It will be the doctor's responsibilty to examine clients, eg. when fitness to travel is in doubt and high-risk travellers who have a chronic or existing disease which may interfere with or be aggravated by travel.

Pre-travel health questionnaire

A standardised pre-travel health questionnaire can be completed by the patient on arrival at the clinic. Information, such as the patients's age, sex, medical history, current medications, immunisation status and allergic history should be obtained. A note should also be made of the destination, planned excursions, season of travel, travel routes and specific risks to which a patient could be exposed. The questionnaire should include details of:

▼ destination

▼ duration of journey

▼ mode of travel

▼ season of travel

▼ holiday type

▼ functional ability

▼ medical status

▼ propensity to travel sickness

▼ visual acuity

▼ hearing ability

▼ vaccination status

▼ insurance cover

▼ travel phobias and anxieties

▼ current medication.

By filling in the questionnaire, responses can be scored as low, medium or high risk and the traveller who is at high health risk can be identified and offered pre-travel advice.

Contraindications to travel should be considered. These could include the effects of travel-related illness, pre-existing disease and/or medication. Around fiveper cent of travel-related disease is vaccine-preventable. Although potential travellers should receive appropriate vaccinations, health may be better protected by adopting a sensible lifestyle, taking preventative measures and being aware of the potential health risks endemic at the chosen destination.

A standardised questionnaire protocol

Demographic details	Risk		
	Low	Med	High
Age: 65–74	*		
75–85		*	
85+			*
Destination			
Western Europe/Canada/North America/New Zealand/Australia	*		
Eastern Europe/The former Eastern Block/Mediterranean Littoral		*	
Tropics/South East Asia/India/Far East/Asia			*
Season			
Favourable	*		
Inclement/monsoon		*	
Transport mode			
Air		*	
Sea	*		
Land	*		
Travel duration			
Short	*		
Long haul		*	
Holiday type			
Visit to relatives/city tours	*		
Safari/Up-Country/Adventure/Sporting			*
Climate			
Moderate/low altitude	*		
Climatic extremes/high altitude			*
Smoking status			
Non smoker	*		
Smoker		*	
Functional disability			
None	*		
Pre-existing functional defect		*	
Incontinence		*	
Psychological disturbance			
Stable personality	*		
Phobia/confusional state/anxiety		*	

Demographic details	Risk		
	Low	Med	High
Predisposition to motion sickness			
Absent	*		
Definite		*	
Current physical status			
Healthy	*		
Moderately healthy		*	
Poor health			*
Pre-existing chronic disease			
Absent	*		
Renal and hepatic disease		*	
Cardiovascular disease, cerebrovascular disease		*	
Diabetes — non insulin dependent		*	
Diabetes — insulin dependent			*
Chronic obstructive airways disease (vital capacity <50%)			*
Epilepsy		*	
AIDS			*
Current mental status			
Normal	*		
Disturbed/diminished			*
Visual acuity			
Normal	*		
Diminished		*	
Auditory function			
Severe deafness		*	
Vaccination status			
Full protection	*		
Absent, no previous vaccinations			*
Special considerations			
Terminal illness			*
Potential medical facilities			
North Europe/New Zealand/Australia/North America	*		
Africa/Asia		*	
Up-Country or remote destinations			*
Insurance			
Adequate	*		
Exclusion clauses		*	
No insurance of any kind			*

Management plan

Creating a customised management plan can minimise potential risks. This plan should:

1. Evaluate risk using a questionnaire (see *Appendix I*).
2. Advise patients of their current risk status
3. Identify factors which can be changed to decrease risk
4. Provide adequate vaccination and prophylaxis
5. Provide adequate advice about precautions that can be taken en route
6. Counsel on appropriate changes in drug medication
7. Give advice to minimise the effects of pre-existing disease while abroad and en route.

Appropriate certificates and referral letters should be supplied and certificates required by transport authorities or tour operators should be completed. Advice should be given on where to obtain travel health education information booklets.

Advice

Pre-travel health counselling by a nurse is effective in reducing the incidence of medical consultations both when travelling and on return to the UK (McIntosh *et al*, 1994).

Travel advice should be relevant, accurate, practical and tailored to the individual (Reed *et al*, 1995). It should not become a major hindrance to enjoyment of the holiday. Consultations should be carefully structured and it should be remembered that the most numerous and serious health problems abroad are the result of trauma and road traffic accidents, particularly in the young. In older age groups, the most common incidents arise from underlying chronic disorders, such as myocardial and cerebrovascular ischaemia and chronic pulmonary disease. Infections may be serious and even fatal but are not the most common adverse effects of travel.

Education and instruction leaflets

Precautionary advice from the nurse and doctor can be reinforced by written instruction leaflets. Typical examples cover:

▼ avoidance of contaminated water

▼ dangers of infected food and its avoidance

▼ adverse effects of ultraviolet light

▼ health hazards of long haul flights.

▼ adverse effects of high altitude

▼ risks of accident and trauma

▼ malaria prophylaxis and prevention

▼ hepatitis and HIV infection.

Leaflets can supplement and reinforce the advice given by a nurse or doctor, but are not as beneficial if given without professional counselling (McIntosh *et al*, 1995).

Information database

Information must be accurate and access to a computerised database, such as TRAVAX should be arranged by the clinic. This can be made available to medical practitioners and nurses through a modem and computer. Data is available from the Scottish Centre for Infection and Environmental Health (SCIEH) in Glasgow and other UK centres.

Travellers should be reminded that medical facilities in inaccessible places, even in Europe, may not reach the standard of those available at home. Travel to medical facilities may mean a journey of many miles over poor roads or tracks, and emergency care may be hours or even days away. Local facilities are frequently limited, with a lack of medical and nursing expertise and poorly maintained or inadequate equipment. Non-disposable equipment is still used in many developing nations and in much of the former Soviet Republic. There is, therefore, a risk of blood-borne infection from contaminated needles, intravenous and infusion materials.

Travellers do not always appreciate the importance of medical insurance cover while abroad. It may be purchased as part of the travel 'package' and the small print exclusions often render the cover worthless. Many people with a pre-existing illness will have to pay an extra premium for adequate cover and further premiums are payable by the old who are often excluded from standard agreements. The value of the cover purchased needs to be carefully assessed. The cost of repatriation and care in places, such as the United States, can be prohibitively expensive. It should also be remembered that medical facilities may be non-existent. However well-insured the traveller is, protection will be illusory and count for nothing. Emergency services, however good or expensive, are irrelevant if patients die before they can be reached.

Immunisation

Immunisation protocols are available for the travel health nurse and he/she should use these to ensure that the traveller only receives vaccinations appropriate to the destination of choice. Cholera vaccinations are still occasionally given to travellers despite World Health Organization recommendations that they are ineffective and unnecessary (WHO, 1992).

Some immunisations have side-effects which make their use inadvisable in the chronically ill and the very old. Many vaccinations are contraindicated in pregnancy and in very young children. Yellow fever immunisation has, until recently, only been available in a few registered centres but changes to the regulations now allow general practices to apply for recognition as yellow fever centres. This is a potential source of income for such practices, as the geographical area covered is usually wide and practices that are not registered will refer their own patients for vaccination.

General advice

Infected water and food are common sources of disease, so advice on how to avoid these infections is important. Water sterilising tablets and equipment, such as the 'Travel Well' can be sold by travel clinics. Travellers should be advised about skin damage caused by sunburn. Its potential carcinogenic effects should be mentioned and advice on protection should be given. There are risks from insect bites; malaria, leishmaniasis, schistosomiasis and onchocerciasis. Bilharzia can be contracted from fresh water in the Nile, Lakes Victoria and Malawi and in the Kariba Dam. These are all areas that are frequently visited by tourists and leaflets and advice should be made available through the travel clinic.

Psychological stresses of travel are a source of distress for the anxious traveller. Physiological disorders can affect elderly people who find themselves trying to manoevre heavy luggage down escalators, or walking to aircraft parked at a terminal some distance from their original setdown point. Clients should be warned about the effects of extremes of temperature and exposure to high altitude. Incontinence can be a problem for some travellers and tactful questioning or completing the questionnaire on risk assessment can aid diagnosis and the tailoring of suitable advice.

High risk

People at high risk are those who are pregnant, the elderly, backpackers, voluntary service workers travelling to rural areas and those living in rural parts of the country. Further advice concerning the additional risks to which they may be exposed should be proffered. Special attention must be given to those with pre-existing illness, such as chronic bronchitis, asthma, diabetes, myocardial and cerebrovascular ischaemia, Parkinson's disease and AIDS. Advice should also be given to travellers accompanied by children, with specific advice on how to treat diarrhoea and vomiting and how to avoid dehydration.

Risks after return

Travel clinics have the responsibility of identifying travellers and notifying health officials if clients are suffering from an illness with the potential to cause a public health hazard. Returning travellers could, potentially, infect other members of their family and their colleagues at work. Health and childcare workers and food handlers will need to be issued with a certificate to sign them off work. Those with suspected food poisoning or dysentery will require stool sampling and laboratory investigation. Dysentery, viral hepatitis, typhoid and malaria are all notifiable diseases and must be reported to the local health authority. Staff will also need to treat patients still suffering from diseases contracted abroad and which have not responded to previous treatment from overseas medical professionals. In a patient presenting with pyrexia of unknown origin, the possibility of malaria must always be considered.

Information sources

Travel health clinics can access data from tropical disease units and scientific journals. The International Society of Travel Medicine holds biennial conferences where travel health issues are discussed in depth. The British Travel Health Association also has an annual conference and educational meeting. Travel Medicine International journal, which is produced bimonthly, is another source of relevant information.

Conclusion

Demands for health advice and vaccination for travelling to other countries has encouraged the growth of general practitioner and commercial travel health clinics. Such clinics allow nurses and doctors to assess the health risks of travellers, identifying specific health risks related to their destination, mode of travel and itinerary. They are there to provide a source of informed health advice and give the traveller information about possible risks, as well as providing the opportunity to assess their effectiveness in preventing and reducing the incidence of travel-acquired disease.

Travel agents are now compelled by EC regulation, to offer appropriate health advice to intending travellers and many will do this by referring clients to general practitioners and clinics. Travel-related illnesses can be reduced by ensuring that proper advice, appropriate vaccination, prophylaxis and counselling are given by qualified professionals who can tailor their responses to meet the individual's needs.

References

Dupont HL, Steffen R (1997) Travel medicine as a unique specialty. In: *Textbook of Travel Medicine and Health*. Decker Publishing, Hamilton

McIntosh I (1995) Setting up a general practice health clinic. *Trav Med Int* **13**: 148–51

McIntosh I, McPherson H (1993) The impact of travel-acquired illness on the primary care service at home and abroad. *Scott Med* **13**:15

McIntosh I, Reed J, Power K (1994) Travel-acquired illness, the world traveller and the family doctor and the need for pre-travel education. *Scott Med J* **39**: 40–4

Reed J, McIntosh I, Power K (1995) Travel illness and the family practitioner. *J Trav Med* **4**: 192–7

Tilley H (1997) The role of the nurse in travel clinics. *Trav Med Int* **15**: 19–22

World Health Organization (1992) *International Travel and Health*. HMSO, London

2

Land travel trauma and the vacationer

Many travellers, travel agents and some medical advisers believe that infectious disease is the most common health hazard to affect the travellers (Keystone *et al*, 1994). However, trauma is more common, with infections representing only a small proportion of the medical complaints suffered by globe-trotters (Fairhurst, 1994). Much of health promotion and prophylaxis is directed at infectious diseases which are endemic in tropical or developing countries. Little consideration is given to the risk to health from trauma, although this is an important cause of death in global travellers.

Trauma

Table 2.1: Percentage of trauma mortality in all deaths related to international travel

Study by	N	Date	%
Sniezek	17988	1991	23.0
Hargarten	2463	1991	22.0
Prociv	421	1995	26.0
Paixio	952	1991	20.7

About one third of travel insurance claims are the result of accidental injury to the insured (Department of Health, 1995). They are often alcohol related and have been identified as the main cause of death in younger travellers abroad (Paixio, 1991). Use of preventative strategies to diminish risks could perhaps prevent many of these incidents. Many infectious diseases are preventable and tourists accept vaccination as a means of protection. Protective programmes should also be adopted to reduce foreseeable trauma risks. Many travellers fail to maintain the commonsense care they take at home to avoid accidents, and rarely consider what additional precautions might be appropriate to their holiday or business destination.

Road transport-related trauma

Road transport always poses some danger to users, especially those who are careless or ignorant of local conditions. A World Health Organization report in 1993 (WHO, 1993) revealed that road traffic accidents (RTA) are one of the leading causes of mortality in travellers. Greater awareness of risk could ensure that safety precautions are observed. Most transport risks can be minimised if common sense is used.

Conventional measures to protect against disease are important. However, travel health clinic staff should place more emphasis on advising travellers of the risks to health of ignoring simple safety precautions. Advice on accident prevention has the potential to considerably reduce morbidity. Travellers are frequently overwhelmed by new cultures and unaware that safety regulations and legislation may fail to meet the criteria they are used to in the UK. Carried away by holiday euphoria or over indulgence in alcohol or drugs, many people fail to observe even basic caution.

Clients with physical disabilities and the victims of accidents often require expensive evacuation. Repatriated, they may place a heavy burden on health service resources. Multiple trauma caused by RTA is the most common reason for air medical evacuations (Rose, 1990). In a review of pathologies requiring medical evacuation (Boutineau 1994), 34% were the result of trauma and road traffic accidents were most common.

Fairhurst (1994) reporting on 1369 consecutive medical problems advised by foreign travellers, found 30.9% were due to trauma and only 1.7% to tropical or exotic infections. Two years later, a further sample of 30% reported trauma as a presenting feature. These were predominantly falls, sports injuries and RTAs. In a survey of medically assisted repatriated travellers, 40.5% were due to trauma (Obadia and Vilotojevic, 1994).

Accidents are a major source of avoidable disability and death in the UK, especially in those under 30 years of age. Road traffic accidents are the most common source of injury although they have been reduced by safety measures, such as safety belts, motor cycle helmets, annual vehicle roadworthiness tests, improved vehicle safety design and inflation bags. The ratio of risk to road users in Britain, using heavy goods drivers as 1, is 2.5:1 for car drivers, 3.1:1 for cyclists and 60:1 for motor cyclists (Bewes, 1993). Preventive measures, common in the UK, do not exist in many of the countries visited by tourists and businessmen. A third of British traffic travels on motorways which are safer than non-segregated traffic routes (Road Traffic Statistics, 1996). In the UK, drivers are used to travelling on the opposite side of the road to most countries abroad. For all these reasons, and because speed enforcement laws are less rigorously applied, the risk of experiencing an RTA is significantly greater.

The percentage of RTA deaths to all trauma-related mortality (International Travel) %		
Sniezek and Smith (1991) 37	Hargarten (1991) 27	Prociv (1995) 28

The association beween RTAs and alcohol consumption is well recognised and the availability of cheap alcohol in many countries visited by tourists is an additional risk. Hired car, coach and taxi drivers, as well as other road users may have been drinking before driving. As drink and drive regulations and enforcement vary (Colon, 1985), the risks of RTA also vary. Economically undeveloped countries with poor, heavily congested road systems have a higher risk. In some developing countries, RTA fatality rates have increased rapidly, with Kenya, Sabah, St. Lucia and Zambia showing more than 100% increase over a 10-year period. Nairobi has a thirty-five percent and Indonesian cities a hundred and forty percent higher accident rate than similar cities in the UK (Jacobs and Fouracre, 1977). Information about non-fatal motor vehicle accidents and tourist and traveller injury is difficult to obtain and poorly recorded in the literature (Hargarten, 1991a). Tourists are hospitalised and ultimately return to their own countries. Most do so on commercial flights without a central record of their experience.

India has 1% of the world's vehicles and 6% of all road accidents. RTAs and resultant deaths and injuries have increased in India by an average of 8% annually in recent years and 25% of all bus accidents occur there (Tinker, 1997). A drive along the Great Trunk Road is an experience few travellers wish to repeat. The road is narrow, elevated, skirted by deep ditches, grossly congested with trucks, coaches, buses, cyclists, pedestrians, pack animals, stray cows and camels. Sikh truck drivers hug the middle of the road in defiance of other road users. Vehicles are often unroadworthy, drivers over-tired or on drugs. At night, unlit transport, people and animals cause death, injury and chaos, and burnt out transport, victim of RTA, litters the roadside.

This picture is common on many roads in developing Asia, Africa and South America. The Asian Pacific region with relatively few vehicles and roads, accounts for half of vehicle-related deaths. Depending upon the developing country and the region, the death/ serious injury rate can be 20–70 times higher than in developed countries.

Death rates for accidents per 10,000 motor vehicles are 2–3 for many near European countries and the USA, 28 for Mexico and 54 for Guatamala (USNSC, 1986). In a study in Mexico, 17% of all deaths of US citizen travellers were due to motor vehicles (Guptill *et al*, 1990). Increased trauma risk for travellers is due to:

- ▶ inadequate legislation or legislation that is not enforced
- ▶ a lack of properly policed roads and vehicle regulations
- ▶ unfamiliar or hazardous environments
- ▶ lack of or inadequate health and safety regulations
- ▶ poorly maintained, unmarked, unlit, unmade and badly built roads
- ▶ badly maintained or old vehicles without safety devices that are not tested for roadworthiness
- ▶ bicycles, animals and pedestrians on congested roads
- ▶ unlicensed, untested drivers and those under the influence of alcohol and drugs
- ▶ hired, unfamiliar vehicles.

Traffic accidents in foreign countries are the most common cause of death in Peace Corps volunteers (Hargarten and Baker, 1985) and American missionaries (Frame, 1992). Dutch workers in developing countries have a mortality rate double that of the population living in Holland with RTAs being the principal cause. When adjustment is made for the number of registered vehicles, the RTA fatality rate is 20 times higher in Ethiopia, Kenya and Botswana than in Europe (Dessie *et al*, 1991). Drivers are often young, inexperienced males. The proportion of pedestrians injured is greater in these countries than in developed countries where a higher proportion of injuries and deaths occur to vehicle occupants.

Many under-developed countries are undergoing rapid industrialisation and a consequent increase in the amount of road transport. In China motor vehicle registrations are growing at a rate of 20% per year, whereas in the UK in 1995, motor traffic increased by 2% (Road Traffic Statistics, 1996). Annual road deaths in China are approximately 50,000 and road trauma is a major health problem. Road death rates are already close to those in the USA but the Chinese road fatality epidemic is just beginning. Currently there are five vehicles per thousand on Chinese roads compared to 770 on US roads. When vehicles, cycles and pedestrians mingle there is traffic chaos and injury.

Tourists in their deluxe coaches are not insulated from the turmoil of traffic commonly found in many national capitals. These cities are on the itinerary of many international coach companies. Coach drivers can be unskilled, over-worked, on drugs or under the influence of drink.

Case histories

> *I was driven along the narrow, truck-congested road between Istanbul and the Mediterranean by a coach driver who had been driving constantly for ten hours. He was high on hashish and insisted on driving with his feet on the steering wheel, until forcibly removed from his seat by terrified passengers.*
>
> *On another occasion in Nicaragua, the coach driver had been quietly drinking alcohol over the lunch break. His performance on the road in the afternoon was erratic and accompanied by frenzied bursts of singing and waving his hands in the air. He failed to negotiate a turning. The bus smashed into a bridge which wrecked the coach, injuring some of the passengers.*
>
> *An even more fear-provoking journey occurred in Bhutan which has only recently built its first roads and has few cars and very young drivers. The latter vie with one another in death defying journeys along precipitous narrow roads. Our driver tried to copy his compatriots who had squeezed past an Indian army munitions convoy. He underestimated the gap beween a truck full of ammunition and nearly blew the minibus*

up as it scraped the length of the truck. Sparks flew into the air as metal scraped against metal, until he eventually hit a large boulder and came to an abrupt stop. Passengers' complaints to the senior driver, conditioned to such reckless driving, brought only an amused response.

Tourists are unrealistically careless about their vulnerability to accidents when travelling by road overseas. This is even more remarkable when compared to fears about air travel. In a large survey few people admitted to anxieties about road travel but 20% suffered from anxieties about flying (McIntosh *et al*, 1996). Yet flying is a particularly safe form of transport with only one accident reported per half a million flights. According to Trevarthen (1995) the chance of being killed in an RTA is 1000 times greater than in a flying accident.

Risk of fatal air accidents compared to other transport and occupations
4 times more likely travelling by bus
8 times more likely when walking
8 times more likely in a boating accident
10 times more likely at work

Tourists hire, cars, minibuses, beach buggies, four-wheel drive vehicles, motor cycles, scooters, bicycles and horses. Choice is usually determined by price rather than by safety features. They choose vehicles they would never consider for their personal transport at home. They accept four-wheeled vehicles without seat belts, air bags or road test and ride two-wheeled transport without helmets or protective clothing. These travellers are at high personal health risk. Improved risk education by health professionals, staffing travel clinics could modify the travelling public's distorted awareness of their personal vulnerability. Higher risk groups should be given specifically targeted advice about the possibility of an RTA when abroad.

High risk road users

Children on bicycles and young adults hiring cars, motor cycles, mopeds, scooters and cycles have high accident rates. The elderly are at particular risk. Older drivers find it more difficult to judge the speed, intentions and directions of other road users. They are more likely to have problems with a different environment if driving an unfamiliar vehicle in another country. In 1989 21% of all car drivers killed on roads in the UK were over 60 years of age and the risk of fatality or serious injury increases with age (Department of Transport, 1991).

Young adults are more likely to drive under the influence of drink when abroad, are less likely to wear helmets on bicycles or motor bicycles and often fail to check the roadworthiness of hired vehicles. Children, unaccustomed to different road rules and at play, are also more likely to become casualties in unfamiliar surroundings (Agran and Winn, 1993).

Pedestrian accidents

Fatal and non-fatal pedestrian accidents are also an increased risk for the international traveller. In elderly travellers, deafness, confusion, slower reflexes and loss of agility increases the accident rate (Department of Transport 191). Pedestrian accident rates in Sweden and Holland are a third less than in the USA, whereas in Portugal and Greece they are 1.5 times greater (Hargarten *et al*, 1991), and in cities of the third world, rates are much higher. Inattention, unfamiliarity with the locality, traffic flow, transport regulations, language constraints and careless driving are all contributory causes.

Emergency assistance

If the traveller is involved in an RTA, he/she may be treated promptly at the scene of the accident by doctors or paramedics and taken without delay to an effective accident and emergency unit with intensive care facilities. However, good trauma care systems may be some distance from the scene of the accident, even in developed countries. Geography may present obstacles to the speed and quality of care available (O'Keefe *et al*, 1994).

Case history

> *Barrie (1994) recounts the history of a motor cyclist overtaking a taxi and colliding head-on with a truck in rural Jamaica. Prompt medical aid was not readily available. Transport to a clinic with poor facilities was only possible after the taxi driver was paid to make a detour.*

Insurance cover is only partly protective and only as good as the proximity of facilities, their quality and that of their staff. Hospitals can be far away and lack modern equipment, medication and trained staff. Inadequate emergency medical treatment at the site of the incident, particularly cardio-respiratory resuscitation, and inadequate hospital facilities are common in many areas of the world. In a study of road traffic accidents in New Delhi, it took more than 15 minutes to transport 85% of the patients to hospital and only 4% were transported by ambulance. The rest were transported in a service bus full of passengers.

Inadequate prehospital care has been highlighted as the cause of a 2.5 times higher mortality rate in cases of serious head injury, in intensive care centres in India against the rate of that in the USA (Colohan *et al*, 1989). Blood for transfusion may not be readily available or what is available may be contaminated. HIV infection and post transfusion hepatitis are possible risks in developing countries (Desai, 1993). In many parts of the world, well equipped services are not available. Severely injured RTA victims cannot supervise the quality of care or the sterility of the equipment and blood products which are used in their treatment.

Considerations which travel clinic staff should highlight, include:

▶ hire of roadworthy vehicles

▶ hire of vehicles with safety features

▶ avoid driving on unlit and unmade roads after dark in undeveloped countries

▶ possibility of a contaminated blood transfusion in the case of accident

▶ scarcity of casualty facilities

▶ the necessity for adequate insurance protection and recognition that this can be compromised by a lack of skills in local health professionals, inadequate medical facilities or casualty evacuation

▶ dangers of driving when suffering from jet-lag (Horne and Reyner, 1996)

▶ passengers should take into account the risks of fatigue, alcohol and drug misuse, and a lack of driving skills in their transport drivers. They should refuse to be driven by such individuals

► travelling in monsoon conditions or during inclement weather should be avoided if possible.

Case history

> *When travelling on the Karakorum Highway, the highest, major public road in the world, which runs from Pakistan to China, the monsoon arrived early. The journey was punctuated by mudslides, rockfalls, avalanches and floods and the bus was inadequately supplied with emergency and survival gear. Passengers were forced to clear boulders and rubble from stretches of road. Vehicles were caught between falling rocks, blocking the road in front and behind. Passengers spent two days and nights in unheated vehicles, at high altitude with little food or protective clothing. They were fortunate to survive.*

Avoidable injuries place unnecessary burdens on state resources. The travel industry and travel clinic personnel should ensure that tourists and businessmen are aware of the risks and encouraged to observe sensible precautions to reduce such risks (McKee, 1996). Guidance on how to travel safely may save more lives than the campaigns currently in place to promote vaccination or prophylactic treatment when clients are abroad.

Hiring transport

Advice for international travellers on safe driving

► avoid alcohol on driving days

► avoid driving at night in developing countries

► hire cars from reputable companies

► test drive the vehicle before hiring, checking brakes, steering and safety aids

► use seat belts in cars and a helmet on motor cycle or scooter

► check that your driver has not been taking alcohol or drugs

► avoid riding in the back of pick-up trucks

► do not hire a vehicle in which you would not be prepared to ride at home

► remember that if you have an accident, emergency aid may be distant, and depend on the skills and resources of the nearest doctor and nurse. These skills and resources may be limited

► accident insurance is only as effective as the availability and quality of the local emergency and evacuation service

► avoid driving when suffering from jet-lag.

References

Agran F, Winn D (1993) The bicycle, a developmental toy versus a vehicle. *J Pediatr* **91**: 752–5

Barrie M (1994) Road crash, smashed paradise. *Mon Week* July 31

Bewes PC (1993) Trauma and accidents. *Br Med Bull* **49**(2): 454–64

Boutineau (1994) Pathologies in medical evacuation. Paper. *Third International Conference of the International Society of Travel Medicine*, Paris

Colohan AR, Alves WM, Gross CR *et al* (1989) Head injury mortality in 2 centres with different emergency medical centres. *J Neurosurg* **71**: 201–7

Colon I (1985) The role of tourism in alcohol related highway fatalities. *Int J Addict* **20**: 577–81

Department of Health (1995) *Health Information for Overseas Travel*. HMSO, London

Department of Transport (1991) *The Older Road User*. DoT, London

Dessie T, Larson P (1991) Motor vehicle injuries in Addis Abeba. *J Trop Med Hyg* **94**: 395–500

Fairhurst RJ (1994) Accidents and travellers. *J Trav Med* **12**(4): 161

Frame JD, Lange R *et al* (1992) Mortality trends of American missionaries in Africa. *Am J Trop Med* **42**: 686–90

Guptill KS, Hargarten S, Baker T (1990) American travel deaths in Mexico. *West J Med* **154**: 169–71

Hargarten S (1991) International travel and motor vehicle crash deaths. *Trav Med Int* **9**: 106–10

Hargarten SW, Baker SP (1985) Fatalities in the Peace Corps. *JAMA* **10**: 1326–9

Hargarten SW, Baker TD, Guptill K (1991) Overseas fatalities of US citizens travellers. *Am J Emerg Med* **20**: 622–6

Horne JA, Reyner LA (1996) Sleep related vehicle accidents. *Br Med J* **310**: 579–80

Jacobs GD, Fouracre PR (1977) *Supplementary Report 2*. Transport and Road Research Laboratory, Crowthorne, Berkshire

Keystone J, Dismukes R *et al* (1994) Inadequacies in health recommendations provided for international travellers by North American health advisers. *J Trav Med* **1**: 72–8

McIntosh I, Power K *et al* (1996) Prevalence,intensity and sex differences in travel related stressors. *J Int Trav Med* **3**: 96–102

McKee M (1996) Travel associated illness. *Br Med J* **312**: 925–6

Obadia E, Vilotojevic B (1994) Medical repatriation of 853 patients: Pathologies and repatriation methods. Paper. *Third International Conference of the International Society of Travel Medicine*, Paris

O'Keefe Grant E, Hamilton S (1994) Motor vehicle related deaths in Northern Alberta. *J Roy Coll Phys Surg* **27**: 149–52

Paixio M (1991) What do Scots die of abroad? *Scott Med J* **3**: 114–6

Prociv P (1995) Deaths of Australian travellers overseas. *Med J Aust* **163**: 27–30

Road Traffic Statistics (1996) Great Britain and London Traffic Monitoring Report. *Br J Ass Immed Care* **19**: 4–7

Rose S (1990) *International Travel Health Guide*. Travel Medicine Inc. New York

Sniezej JE, Smith SM (1991) Injury mortality among Non US residents in the US 1979–84. *Int J Epidem* **19**: 255–9

Tinker J (1997) Synopsis of the road travel report for India. *Trav Med Int* **15**: 211–2

Trevarthen FD (1995) Flying isn't dangerous but . . . *Trav Med Int* **13**(2): 62–5

United States National Safety Council (1986) *Death Rates For Motor Vehicle Crashes*. NSNCC, Washington (DC)

World Health Organization (1993) *International Travel and Health*. WHO, Geneva

3

Health and safety in the air

In the early days of air travel it was as easy to board an aeroplane as it was to board a coach. Although technical failures often caused delays, aircraft were small. The main safety concern was aircraft-overload and passengers were weighed as well as luggage. Currently, preboarding procedures emphasise hazards associated with air travel. The occasional crash with the loss of life attracts much adverse publicity.

Catastrophic mechanical aircraft failure is rare and aeroplanes are now much safer. Thousands of flights depart daily from international airports and land safely, but still many people have phobias about flying. One in ten adults report an intense fear of flying and 20% of the UK population admit to anxieties strong enough to prevent them from flying. Fear of flying was the second most common travel-related phobia reported in a survey of travellers and non-travellers (McIntosh, 1996). A minority never leave the UK because of a psychological inability to fly in an aircraft. They perceive flying as unsafe.

How rational is this fear of flying? Phobias are involuntary, irrational fears, but people with these fears may be making a realistic appraisal of the dangers of this travel mode. Air crashes are widely reported in the media. This encourages a phobic reaction in some people, which might legitimately be considered a protective reaction to exposure to a potentially dangerous situation. Flying confronts several innate fears, such as fear of heights, falling, enclosed spaces and social crowding (Greco, 1989). Airlines, however, produce statistics suggesting that the most dangerous element in international air transit is the car drive to the airport.

Flying safety

The overall air accident rate per trip was 50 per million in 1960 and is one per million today. The accident rate per kilometre is also lower than it was 20 years ago. When measured in terms of deaths per distance travelled, air travel appears a safe mode of transport, but statistics are skewed by the huge distances travelled safely. Airlines quote figures of one accident per 500,000 miles. Comparatively, the risk of being killed is eight times greater when walking or boating, ten times greater at work and 1000 times greater in a road accident (Trevarhen, 1995). However, if fatality rate per man hour of exposure is calculated, car and air travel appear equally hazardous.

Air accident fatalities

World-wide, airline flying accounts for an average 1100 lives lost per annum and the aviation industry points reassuringly to this safety record. However, as air traffic volumes continue to increase, the number of crashes is likely to rise. Passenger volumes have been increasing by 6% annually and projections suggest inexorable growth over the next decade with aeroplanes of increased capacity. The US Federal Aviation Administration (USFAA) has warned that major aircraft losses are likely with the global increase in flights. Boeing Corporation and USFAA forecast that improvements in aircraft safety records are coming to an end (Economist Leader, 1997).

There were 944 aircraft accident-related deaths in 1987 and 1840 in 1996 with a 25% increase in casualties in the last three years. The volume of air travel has increased by a third in that period, but may double by the year 2010. At current accident rates, that would certainly infer there could be more crashes. Air travel has risen eight-fold since the sixties and there are now 15 million large jet flights annually, carrying 1.3 billion people across the world.

Causes of crashes

mechanical failure	pilot error
inadequate air traffic control	the use of ageing aeroplanes
over-dependence on cockpit computers	
terrorism	acts of war

Pilot error accounts for about 70% of accidents. Confusion between whether the pilot or a flight management system was in control occurred in 24 recent serious accidents. Inadeqate air traffic control over parts of Asia, Africa and the Pacific has been criticised by the International Federation of Airline pilots (IFALPA).

The average age of half the world fleet of 1000 jumbo airliners is 18.8 years, a worrying trend. The accident rate for freight aircraft, many of which are elderly, is much higher than for passenger planes. Developing countries have a reputation for less safe air travel. For example, the former USSR had an average of six major accidents in the 1980–90 period and 12 in 1996.

The majority of commercial aircraft crashes result from pilot error with some labelled 'controlled flight into terrain' when the plane has been flown into a mountain. Accidents rarely occur during the cruising phase of a flight, other than in explosive incidents. They occur primarily on take off and landing, although these procedures only account for 6% of flight time.

The aircraft industry's objective is to ensure that no more than one fatal accident occurs in multicrew aircraft per 10 million miles flown, with only a tenth of these accidents due to air crew incapacitation. A further aim is that on-board safety critical systems may only fail once per thousand million miles flying and be implicated in a crash once per several million flights (Trevarthen, 1995).

Statistics on safety fault violations and near misses are closely guarded by airline authorities but are highly pertinent to flight safety. These statistics should be communicated to a wider audience with provision of safety leagues tables, so that passengers can be more aware of the travel risks associated with certain carriers.

Panic attacks in air-borne passengers are the most frequent events reported to air crew. Passengers, who have steeled themselves for the flight despite anxieties over travel safety, have ample time to sit and consider their strange environment, possible engine malfunction, hijack, terrorist explosion and incarceration in a closed tube speeding through the skies.

Realistically, aeroplanes rarely hurtle uncontrolled from high altitude. However, a fuel or bomb explosion can rip apart an airliner, killing all the passengers.

Case history

When PanAm 103 blew up near Lockerbie in 1988, the plane split apart. People in the rear section were suddenly exposed to an icy blast and wind forces of over 130mph which stripped off clothing. Air pressure plummeted from a cabin pressure equivalent of 2500m altitude to equal that at the cruising height of 12,000m, about a quarter that at sea-level. Internal body organ gases expanded to four times normal. Expanding gases caused the lungs to swell then collapse. With tornado force winds filling the cabin, breathing became impossible for most and passengers lost consciousness. Passengers were bombarded with cabin debris and tossed out of the jet to be exposed to crosswinds in an air temperature of 50°F below zero. One or two trapped in the more sheltered nose cone survived a free fall. They were still alive on contact with the ground although they died shortly afterwards (Cox, 1988).

Remarkably, people have survived falls from high flying aircraft. In 1972 a Yugoslav air hostess fell 11,000m after a DC 9 exploded over the Czech Republic. Individuals have also survived the hypothermia experienced at high altitudes. During the Second World War people were regularly flown out of occupied Europe in the unheated bomb bays of mosquito aircraft at some risk to their lives. One eminent scientist fleeing from occupied Norway was hypothermic and unconscious when the plane finally reached Scotland. The planes were relatively low flying, but more recently a 22-year-old Indian survived after spending ten hours in the wheel bay of a Boeing 737 flying at 12,000m from Asia to London. He lived despite exposure to temperatures of minus 60°C but his brother, who was with him, died.

Physiological trauma in flight

Cabin hypoxia

Aircraft mishap is not the only risk to passengers. The pO_2 levels in pressurised jet-liner cabins can be as low as 30–40mm Hg. The physiological trauma associated with flying is a risk for those with cardiac and respiratory disease. In an aircraft cabin pressurised to 1900m altitude, an arterial oxygen saturation of 70mm Hg at sea level is required to maintain adequate in-flight oxygen saturation and anyone with a resting PaO_2 value less than this will have respiratory problems. Exposure to hypoxia during flight is likely to cause adverse cardiopulmonary events in those with compromised health They account for a significant number of in-flight emergencies (Leon *et al*, 1996).

Pressure changes increase the risk of spontaneous pneumothorax in those with blebs and bullae. Changes in blood viscosity bring the risk of deep venous thrombosis — the economy class syndrome (Sahiar and Mohler, 1994), pulmonary embolism and cerebral vein thrombosis (Pfausler *et al*, 1996). Patients with existing congestive cardiac failure or dilated cardiac myopathy are at high risk. Physiological trauma due to air sickness is now rare on high flights in large aircraft.

Physical trauma in flight

Passengers can suffer physical trauma in flight but this is uncommon. Sudden turbulence when people are in the toilets or walking the passages can cause falls, contusions and fractures but wearing a seat belt reduces the possibility of such injury. Severe turbulence has caused overhead storage bins to open and passengers can be struck by falling objects. This is a rare occurrence as most flights fly round or above severe weather.

In-flight illness

Serious in-flight illness is fortunately rare (Roscoe, 1997). On major airlines world wide, the in-flight health-related death rate was 0.31 per million passengers carried or 25 deaths per million aircraft departures over an eight year period (Chapman, 1995). At Los Angeles airport, with 8.5 million arriving passengers in one year, seven had died in-flight. Of the 260 reported medical complaints, about one in 39,000 passengers, only 25 were hospitalised (Speizer *et al*, 1989). One international carrier reported that the on-board medical kit had been opened 362 times over one year, representing a frequency of usage of one in 1900 flights.

Passengers, who are unwell in-flight, often tolerate symptoms until landing.They report to destination hospitals and clinics and thus dilute the statistics for on-board illness. In one study of 754 travellers, a quarter experienced medical problems after the flight and four of the five cardiac arrests occurred within minutes of deplaning. Studies of flight-related health problems are now 5–10 years old with no recent major studies at a time when changing pattens of air travel may have increased health risk (Neumann, 1996).

In-flight medical incidents

Requests for doctors to respond to in-flight medical incidents meet with a medical response in three out of four requests, the majority of incidents not being serious. In the USA, less than one flight per 100,000 is diverted for medical reasons, but flights are relatively short and there is a higher rate on long haul flights. On-board medical kits have limited contents and most clinicians are constrained in their treatment of a patient in need. Space is at a premium and nursing skills are often all that is required until landing.

Acute and increasing abdominal pain with vomiting and collapse may cause a diagnostic dilemma on the ground. In an airborne emergency, a rational, appropriate response, right for patient, passengers and crew, can provoke anxiety for the attending physician, especially if there has to be a route diversion.

Litigation insurance has limitations for the attending physician under such circumstances. According to UK insurance societies: 'Cover is assured for the doctor unless the patient is American, it is an American plane or the plane is landing on US soil'. Most doctors appear to ignore this restriction and offer to help when asked.

Case history

> *I created my own midair medical incident. An unexpected food allergy caused sudden illness followed by unconsciousness in a packed charter Airbus economomy class cabin. Staff were busy with meals and I was the only doctor on board. There was apparently nowhere to lay me flat. I recovered consciousness, bent double over a jump seat in the galley, with meal trays stacked around me and staff stepping over my legs. A glance out of the window was far from reassuring, as a flash of white light hit the wing and ran towards the cabin window.*
>
> *I thought my end had come. The plane was pitching about in the middle of a thunderstorm, somewhere over Malta. This was not an experience one would wish to repeat. In this instance, staff were uninterested, had scant knowledge of first-aid and immediate care came from fellow passengers.*

More than 16 million people leave the UK by air each year and a considerable increase in this number is expected over the next decade. Passengers fly further, on longer flights and more frequently. Many travel apprehensively, some resorting to sedatives and alcohol to calm their anxieties. Some with phobias dread the trip and the return, others avoid travelling abroad.

Despite human error and mechanical defect, air travel has a good safety record. Realistically, travellers should not fear air travel, but should treat it the same as travel by car, coach or train. No form of travel is entirely free from risk.

Approximately 50% of the British population who do not travel abroad are constrained by fears concerning safety (McIntosh, 1996). Such travellers can be reassured by travel health professionals. Those suffering from a fear of flying may be treated by behavioural or hypnotherapists who can rationalise such fears, and offer coping strategies which allow clients to travel abroad. There is a greater risk associated with travel on land and in holiday leisure activities than in travel by air.

References

Chapman PJC (1995) In-flight emergencies. *Trav Med Int* **13**: 171–3

Cox M, Foster T (1988) *Their Darkest Day*. Arrow Books, London

Economist Leader (1997) *Economist* Jan 11: 15–16

Greco TS (1989) A cognitive behavioural approach to the fear of flying. *Phob Pract Res J* **2**: 3–15

Leon M, Lateef M *et al* (1996) Cardiology and travel. *J Int Trav Med* **3**: 168–71

McIntosh IB (1996) Identification and management of aircraft phobias. *J Trav Med Int* **14**: 249–52

McIntosh IB, Power K (1996) Prevalence, intensity and sex differences in travel-related stressors. *J Int Trav Med* **3**: 96–102

Neumann K (1996) Breathing on the go. *Trav Med Int* **14**: 189–4

Pfaussler B,Vollert H *et al* (1996) *J Int Trav Med* **3**:137

Sahiar F, Mohler S (1994) Economy class syndrome. *Aviat Space Med* **65**: 957–60

Roscoe AN (1997) In-flight medical emergencies. *Trav Med Int* **15**: 242–6

Speizer C, Rennie CJ, Breton H (1989) Prevalence of in-flight medical emergencies on commercial flights. *Ann Emerg Med* **18**: 26

Trevarthen FD (1995) Flying isn't dangerous but... *J Trav Med Int* **13**: 62–7

4

Sea cruising, trauma and tragedy

Cruise holidays are becoming increasingly popular after a decline in the mid-twentieth century caused by the introduction of cheap air travel. Ships sail throughout the world on short and long cruises. Europe is the second biggest cruise market with 1.3 million passengers annually (Ward, 1997). Destinations include the Caribbean and Mediterranean seas and ships sail the Atlantic, Pacific and Indian Oceans. Although the prerogative of the affluent for many years, out of season price cutting and commercial competition has reduced cruise costs. They now attract passengers from every social class and are particularly attractive to older, retired people. They appear to offer a protected environment with few physical demands, well-suited to the less agile and partially disabled.

Advertisements and brochures emphasise the 24-hour availability of on-board nursing and medical services for those with chronic illness and for those who may suffer ill health during travel. This apparently benign and friendly cruise environment may be illusory. The risk of collision or fire is well appreciated (Velimorivic, 1990), but other on-board risks are poorly documented, although they may be an important consideration for elderly travellers (McIntosh, 1997).

Large numbers of passengers on cruises are over retirement age, and clients over 80 years of age are common on most voyages.

Cruise passenger age (1994)	
60 years and older	29%
40–59 years	36%
others	35%

(Ward 1997)

Several cruise companies target older, retired clients and some have adapted cabins for the use of the physically disabled. Yet cruise ships do not provide a stable environment. Even if fitted with stabilisers, they roll in high seas. This motion can cause travel sickness and affect the activities of passengers on-board. Ship passengers prefer calm seas, but moderate swells and choppy seas are frequent, even in summer.

Good weather rarely lasts throughout a long cruise, but elderly and infirm clients often book such holidays without considering the possible affects of poor weather on their health. Ship passageways are narrow, cabins doorways can be difficult to manoeuvre through, and stairways are steep, especially in ships which are old and ill equipped. Brochures which present enticing pictures of calm seas, sunny climates and spacious decks are inviting but often misleading. For clients who are disabled and need walking aids or wheelchairs, travel clinic professionals must describe the risks of bad weather, inherent in such holidays. Not only minor injuries can result from a fall caused by rolling seas, there is also the risk of fracture to hips or spine. Minor injury is a nuisance, but a fractured hip can be life-threatening if good surgical intervention is not available.

Exclusions from sea travel

Depressed patients
Alcoholics
The blind/very poorly sighted
Unstable asthmatics
Unstable angina patients and the wheelchair dependent (unless special facilities are available)

Management

Medical review of pre-existing disease
Review of current medication
Medical report for the ship's doctor
List of drugs for the ship's doctor

Counselling

Choice of ship/destination
Travel sickness, prophylaxis
On-board risk assessment
Vaccinations including flu vaccination for those over 65 years with cardiac/pulmonary disease

Advice about sea-sickness — avoidance and treatment

Take an antihistamine tablet or apply a transdermal Scopoderm patch 8 hours before starting the voyage
Keep in the fresh air
Fix the eyes on the horizon
Try to keep the head fixed in relation to the body
Sit midships facing along the vessel's length
Lie down if symptoms seem imminent with the head towards the centre of rotation and close the eyes
Take regular sips of water to avoid dehydration

Delay in transporting a patient to hospital care or surgery, anaesthetic and rehabilitative support which is not of high standard can result in serious illness or even death. Ships' infirmaries can only offer first-aid facilities. Specialist care may be several days away by sea and there may be only limited facilities at the next port of call. Rescue helicopters have a limited flying range and emergency evacuation to the UK may be impracticable if there are no local air sevices. Good health insurance cover is of little relevance if the facilities of the nearest land-based hospital are limited or ill-equipped and medical personnel are inadequately trained.

Trauma is a major part of a ship doctor's emergency work (Flanagan, 1998) on ships carrying predominantly older persons. The majority of health problems reported by ships' doctors are in passengers over 65-years-old and female passengers see the ships doctor twice as freqently as men. The most common injuries in passengers are contusions from falls. Fractures are more frequent in passengers than in members of the crew. They are more likely to break a leg than are crew members who suffer more broken arms.

Common passenger injuries (Martinovic, 1997)

► contusion

► laceration

► burns — usually severe sun burn

► fractures

Ships have to meet rigorous fire and damage regulations with the provision of watertight doors. These raise floor elevations in passages and stairways. Door sills which exclude the entry of water are common on many decks. Some may be a foot high, difficult to negotiate and easy to trip over. They are often unobtrusive in cabins, toilets and showers, causing the unwary to trip and fall.

Deck surfaces can be wet, external stairways slippery and steep, gangways unstable and, if seas are high, may be awash. Few passengers anticipate the amount of walking and stair climbing there can be beween cabins, promenade decks and public rooms. Routes can be hazardous in boisterous seas and dangerous in storms. Older ships and passenger liners built many years ago may have design features which interfere with mobility and fewer elevators than newer ships. Grab rails in large hallways, foyers and wide stairs of modern ships may be out of reach, should an unexpected wave cause the ship to roll. On sun decks, deckchairs soon clutter walkways and it is easy to fall over them.

Quays are usually busy with fork-lift trucks and cranes off-loading freight from moored vessels. They are often wet, greasy and littered with debris, an obstacle course for the visually impaired.

Case history

On the first shore landing of a voyage, an elderly couple gingerly descended the gangway, he using a stick and she supported by his steadying hand. They shuffled forward on the quay, eyes on the waiting tour coach and did not see a loop of twine which lay on the ground in front of them. She put first one foot and then the other within the coil. With her next step it looped over her ankles and she fell heavily dragging him with her. He suffered a strained back and bruised buttocks, but she fractured a scaphoid bone and a hip. With blackeyes and a bleeding nose she was disembarked to local Columbian medical care. Facilities were limited and the city was 4 hours away over rough gravel roads. The ambulance was a converted van and she had a very disagreeable ride to hospital, for orthopaedic surgery.

Ships do not always berth beside a quay. They can anchor offshore and passengers are transferred from ship to shore by tender. This tender can be a large passenger-carrying craft, a high-speed launch or the ship's lifeboat. It may be modern, self-righting and covered, but can be obsolete, open and high-sided. Passengers transfer from ship to tender down a ladder which is slung from the ship's side and on to a pontoon. Ship, tender, pontoon and ladder all move with the waves, and are difficult to traverse, even for clients who are active and fit.

Passengers are manually helped by members of the crew from the ship, down the ladder, on to the pontoon and into the tender. The operation is repeated in reverse when the shore jetty is reached and again on return to the ship. This testing exercise for the fit and young is a manoeuvre that the arthritic and the elderly should not be expected to contemplate. However, clients refuse to be intimidated or prevented by disability from going ashore. They descend from the ship, with walking sticks and support frames, taking risks that would be inconceivable at home. Falls, contusions, lacerations and broken bones are frequently associated with these marine transfers.

Annually, 10,000 people now venture to Antarctica in cruise ships. These journeys are expensive, but attract the wealthy and the old. Transfer to tiny, rocky, snow-covered beaches in the White Continent is by small inflatable craft. Although relatively safe in the water, climbing in and out of these tiny boats is potentially hazardous. A heavy wash from another vessel, or waves from an ice floe falling into the water, can capsize the dinghy, throwing its occupants into freezing water. Unless immediately rescued, survival is doubtful.

Older travellers are often partially-sighted, deaf and physically disabled. Their right to travel is not in question, but they and their companions should be aware of the additional risks of cruise holidays. The goodwill of competent partners and crew members is essential if they are to travel safely. It is when this support is compromised, that the risks become apparent.

Case history

A totally blind man on a Caribbean cruise was accompanied by his wife. She fell at the entrance to the boat, badly bruising her thigh and breaking her dominant arm. This was put in a plaster cast and an arm sling by the ship's doctor who told her to rest in bed. She was incapable of helping her husband who had difficulty in finding his way around the new cabin and could not explore the rest of the ship. He found he could not help her with the personal tasks she could no longer manage. The ship's staff were unable to offer further help so the couple spent most of the cruise confined to their cabin.

Risk factors for passenger injury in cruise ships	
advanced years	physical disability
poor vision	wet decks
raised door sills	steep stairs
ship movement	unsuitable footwear, ie.high heels, flip flops
swimming pools	spa pools and their environs
tender transfer	steep gangways
deck impedimenta	large foyers without grab rails
passage protrusions	interrupted deck rails

The blind and visually impaired can find shipboard life a daunting experience. Floor obstructions often carry written warning signs but there are no audible warnings. Steel doors are left open on passageways, deck and wall rails are interrupted. There are open stairwells above steep stairs and sun loungers, ropes and chains obstruct the decks.

Clients who use a stick, tripod or zimmer frame find that the aid can become an encumbrance on a ship. Ladders, gangways, narrow passages and steep stairs need to be negotiated by grasping handrails. Walking aids can often be a hindrance rather than a help.

Drinking too much alcohol is common on cruise ships and a regular cause of falls, tissue and bone damage, particularly in the old with impaired balance. Falling asleep on deck in the tropical sun is inadvisable. Not only do passengers risk severe sunburn, dehydration and stroke, but they can wake up confused, stumble to their feet and fall down the nearest companion way.

Cruise lines, with litigation in mind, are aware of on-board hazards and place appropriate warning signs. Public announcements of the dangers of wet decks in rough weather are made, but not always heard in cabins or by those who are deaf. The crew may try to reduce risk but these hazards are inherent on ships. Passengers, particularly the elderly, appear to expose themselves inadvertently to risk with no thought for possible consequences. During pre-travel consultations, health professionals should draw such dangers to the attention of their clients and proffer advice about sensible safety precautions.

This advice may suggest that certain cruises should not be taken, especially when there is very high risk for physically compromised travellers. There are times when sea travel is contraindicated and certificates of fitness for sea travel should be refused in the interest of the patient and other passengers. Unfit and disabled passengers slow embarkation and disembarking procedures on a cruise ship and threaten speedy evacuation of passengers in an emergency.

With the revival of sea cruises and an increase in the number of the elderly affluent, a corresponding increase in the number of older people taking cruising holidays is likely. Although most will return home in good health, some will be less fortunate and experience on-board trauma. The travel health professional is trained to assess and advise the degree of risk to health of such holidays. By ensuring that the client has advance information, the risks may be minimised and sea travel will be safer.

Recommendations for travel clinic personnel

▼ consider ports of call and their hinterland and appropriate vaccination

▼ consider hazards inherent in ship board travel and advise older people about them

▼ provide an educational leaflet in the clinic with details of potential cruise ship hazards

▼ be prepared to refuse certificates of fitness for sea travel where this is not in the patients or other passengers best interest

▼ advise potential travellers to choose their ship and itinerary with an eye to their personal safety

▼ ensure that travellers insurance cover is comprehensive .

Educational leaflet for cruise line passengers

● choose your ship and its itinerary carefully to minimise health risk from shipboard hazard

● check number of stairs, elevators, length of passageways, width of foyers

● consider the ports of call and need for immunisation

● what is the access to the shore?

● avoid ship to shore tender operations

● what physical assistance may be made available at embarkation and disembarkation?

● what medical facilities are on board?

● is there X-ray apparatus?

● choose a cabin close to dining and public rooms

● what is the likelihood of severe weather during the cruise?

● be prepared to stay in your cabin and avoid movement around the ship in bad weather

● too much alcohol causes falls and fractures

● do not fall asleep on deck in the tropical sun as this can lead to bad burns, confusion and falls.

References

Flanagan M (1998) Doctor at sea. *Scott Med J* (In Press)

Martinovic N (1997) The morbidity of passengers and crew of the cruiser 'Adriana'. *Trav Med Int* **15**: 194–7

McIntosh I (1997) Health and safety on cruise ships. *Trav Med Int* **15**: 234–7

Velimorivic B (1990) Health hazards of sea tourism. *Trav Med Int* **8**: 69–75

Ward B (1997) *Complete Guide to Cruising and Cruise Ships*. Berlitz, Princeton, N J

5

Winter sports trauma and the traveller

Almost a million Britons take winter sports holidays abroad each year and the majority return without injury. However, careless tourists to snow-covered and mountainous resorts can experience hypothermia, altitude sickness, over-exposure to ultra-violet light radiation, extreme cold and physical injury.

Climbers travel to mountains such as the Himalayas to enjoy adventurous climbing sports. At these altitudes conditions are frequently Arctic. Days are short and climbers may find themselves isolated on icy cliffs, snowy inclines and slippery rocks, in the dark. For the unwary, there is a high risk of falls and deep snow fields on high slopes can result in avalanches. Mountain accidents frequently occur because climbers go too far, too high, too fast and are not prepared to turn back as conditions worsen. Fatigue, makes slips and falls more likely.

Skiers going too fast can lose control and collide with trees or other skiers. Hill trekkers can be at risk of altitude sickness, hostile conditions and climatic extremes. Winter sports novices are inexperienced, sometimes ill-equipped and unprepared for abrupt changes in climatic conditions.

Risks could be reduced if holiday-makers were more aware of them. Travel health clinic professionals should offer pre-travel counselling on potential health hazards and advice on minimising risks. They should tailor advice to meet the individual's needs.

Exposure and hypothermia

Cold climatic extremes expose travellers to the risk of hypothermia, which can kill fit adults within a few hours. Onset is often insidious and climbers are only aware of feeling chilled, numb, lethargic and apathetic. Progress becomes slow and stumbling and there may be some mental confusion. This is followed by incoherence, total confusion, irreversible coma and death if hypothermia is not recognised. The ability to adapt to cold is reduced with increased body surface area to volume ratio. Lean, young rock climbers, teenagers, children and the tall and thin are at extra risk.

What is hypothermia?

Death from cardiac failure-induced hypothermia occurs when the body surface is severely chilled and core temperatures drop sharply.

The condition is divided into mild, moderate and profound hypothermia. In mild hypothermia, core temperatures fall to between 33–35°C, the patient is conscious and experiences feelings of intense cold, strong involuntary shivering and tachycardia. In moderate/profound hypothermia, the core temperature falls below 33°C, a condition which is life-threatening. The shivering reflex disapears below 30°C and ventricular fibrillation or asystole occurs.

Signs and symptoms of exposure

- ▶ unexpected and unreasonable behaviour
- ▶ complaints of coldness and fatigue
- ▶ physical and mental lethargy
- ▶ failure to respond to direct questions or a failure in comprehension
- ▶ abnormal vision
- ▶ slurred speech
- ▶ sudden shivering and fits
- ▶ sudden short bursts of unexpected energy
- ▶ recurrent falls and stumbling
- ▶ disorientation and light-headedness
- ▶ pallor.

Windy, wet and cold conditions are dangerous. Wind speed affects body temperature in cold wet and cold dry conditions. Air temperatures should be assessed as 6°C below ambient temperatures if clothing is wet. Prolonged exposure to cold, high winds, wet clothing or falls into snow or icy water increase the risk of hypothermia (Sneddon, 1993; McIntosh, 1993).

Children, because of their body surface to weight ratio, reduced subcutaneous tissue and immature thermoregulation are more at risk, as are elderly adults who have reduced metabolism, subcutaneous fat and muscle mass. Sweating feet and hands, concurrent infection and recent moderate alcohol intake increase the likelihood of the condition occurring at low ambient temperatures (Roeggla *et al*, 1995).

Severity of hypothermia

Mild	Moderate	Profound
amnesia,apathy,	hallucinations	coma
impaired judgement	loss of consciousness	ventricular fibrillation
increased heart rate	arrythmias	asystole
shivering	shivering stopped	apnoea

Effects of extreme cold

Any person on a winter sports holiday can be affected by low air temperatures. They may suffer from cold collapse (hypothermia), or cold injuries to the skin, such as **frostnip** — minor damage to surface skin when deeper tissues are not affected and rewarming reverses the damage. **Frostbite** is more serious as the deeper tissues freeze due to exposure to cold, and fingers and toes are more likely to be affected. Vasoconstriction and the formation of ice crystals within the tissues are contributory factors and any drop in core temperature increases the risk. Hypoxia, which occurs at high altitude, and the effects of some drug medications are additional risk factors.

Feet and hands are most vulnerable to cold injuries but the ears, nose and cheeks can also be affected. In addition to the ambient temperature, other factors which increase the risk of frostbite are windchill, travelling in open vehicles in windy conditions, failing to use protective oils on exposed skin and failing to wear hats with ear muffs, gloves and scarves (Lehmuscallio *et al*, 1995).

Ultra-violet radiation

Sunburn can be caused by high intensity, ultra-violet radiation. This radiation is common in the thin air conditions of high altitudes. Ultra-violet rays and snow-reflected sunlight affect skiers and mountaineers. Sunlight is divided into ultraviolet B(UVB) (280–315nm) and A(UVB0 (315–400nm). Physiologically, UVB is more dangerous than UVA and is mainly responsible for sunburn, skin ageing, solar keratosis and skin cancer. However, during the middle of the day the amount of UVA reaching the earth's surface is 100 times greater than

UVB. Although higher UVA exposure is necessary to cause sunburn, the risk from this source is high, as the majority of winter sports enthusiasts are in the open at this time of day. It is essential that a sun screen with a high protective factor is used regularly to protect the skin.

Pale-skinned individuals, with fair or red hair and light-coloured eyes are often sun sensitive. Skin can become even more sensitive to sunlight if systemic drugs which cause phototoxic or photoallergic reactions are used. Excessive sunlight can precipitate attacks of herpes simplex eruptions. Children are less likely to take protective measures against sun exposure when skiing and climbing. People over 65-years-old are more likely to develop solar keratosis when exposed to intense sunlight (Verbov, 1994).

Some drugs which may cause phototoxicity

sulphonamides	tetracyclines
nalidixic acid	thiazides
protryptiline	chlorproamazine

Reflected glare from snow fields can cause eye problems, such as conjunctival burns, uveitis and snow-blindness. The ultraviolet light induced conjunctivitis produces painful blepharospasm which can be treated with local anaethetic eye drops. The condition is best avoided by use of snow goggles. Spontaneous recovery is usual once away from sunlight.

The use of of a high SPF sun screen (minimum sun protective factor 15) and eye protection spectacles (BS2724) or wrap round goggles are recommended for winter sports holidaymakers.

Acute mountain sickness (AMS)

Acute mountain sickness is a common condition which can affect any person at high altitude (defined as beyond 2400 metres). The reported prevalence in the European Alps is 9% at 2850m, 13% at 3050m 34% at 3650m, 53% at 4559m (Maggiorini, 1990) and 63% for trekkers in Nepal reaching an altitude of 5400m.

Acute mountain sickness symptoms

headaches	lethargy	altered breathing
nausea	dizzyness	vomiting
disturbed sleep		

Skiers and climbers in the European Alps, the American Rocky Mountains, the Himalayas and the Andes may experience mild symptoms. They become acclimatised if staying and sleeping at lower altitudes. While climbing high by day, climbers to higher altitudes and those who fly to high resorts from low level departure airports are at increased risk from acute mountain sickness.

Almost half of skiers and trekkers flying from low lying airports to 2000m and immediately climbing to 4000m will suffer from AMS. Eighty-four percent of tour trekkers flying to the hotel, Everest View (4205m) developed AMS. American ski resorts are increasingly popular with British skiers and many fly to high ski areas. In one study of nearly 4000 people visiting ski resorts in Colorado, 2000–2880m altitude, 12% suffered three or more symptoms of AMS (Houston, 1985).

It appears that those aged under 20 years are most likely to suffer, possibly because they are too active and ignore warning symptoms. Previous sufferers of AMS are at higher risk, but there are no other certain predictors of vulnerability. Severer forms of AMS appear to be more common in men. Forty-nine men but only one woman were air rescued after suffering from high altitude pulmonary oedema (HAPE), a potentially fatal complication, in a four-year period in the Swiss Alps (Maggiorini, 1990).The approximate incidence of HAPE is 2% in those exposed to high altitude.

Risk factors increase with altitude, especially the sleeping altitude, and the rate of ascent. AMS can be avoided by allowing gradual acclimatisation. A slow graded ascent to higher altitude should be adopted and sleeping accommodation should be as low as possible. Acetazoleamide 250mg per day can be used as a prophylactic beginning at least 24 hours before climbing to an altitude where AMS is a possibility (McIntosh, 1986; Green *et al*, 1981).

HAPE

HAPE is characterised by breathlessness, cough and white frothy sputum which may become bloodstained. Immediate and rapid descent is required if the patient is to survive. In a study of British mountaineers, the fatality rate in high climbers was 4.3%, with 17% due to HAPE. The condition contributed to many of the fatal trauma deaths recorded (Pollard, 1992).

HACE

High altitude cerebral oedema (HACE) is another potentially dangerous condition characterised by severe headaches, irrational behaviour, errors of judgement, hallucinations and ataxia which can rapidly progress to unconsciousness. The victim suffers the symptoms of raised intracranial pressure. Immediate and rapid descent is mandatory if the individual is to survive either of these conditions. Return to a low level altitude will normally reverse milder forms of AMS.

People with cardiopulmonary disease or high blood pressure with possible occlusive arterial disease should seek medical advice or attend a travel health clinic for counselling before travelling to destinations above 4000m. Diabetes mellitis, controlled epilepsy, hypertension and asthma are not contraindications to travelling to high altitude. If an activity holiday is intended, the compounded effects of exercise and high altitude on these conditions should be considered.

Avalanches

Avalanches are a threat to off-piste skiers and winter climbers. They usually occur on steep slopes, on slopes with deep snow or on those where a layer of old snow has been covered by fresh snow. During storms, snow rapidly gathers in gullies and on lee slopes. The crystals are broken down by the wind to form a layer known as windslab. If this lies on top of a less dense layer of snow, it is likely to collapse and trigger an avalanche. Cornices which collapse at the top of gullies also cause avalanches when they hit the slope beneath at speed and with explosive effect. Avalanches also occur when the temperature rises suddenly after fresh snow, so that the melting snow lubricates the layer beneath and slippage occurs.

Types of fatal injury in those caught in an avalanche

crushing	the pressure of snow and ice prevents respiratory chest movements
drowning	dry powder ice invades the lungs and, on melting, the water floods the alveoli
hypothermia	reduced body temperature, leading to a sharp reduction in core temperature and cardiac failure

If the victim survives and is not rescued promptly, hypothermia sets in. Many of the injured suffer trauma to the head sustained during the fall.

Advice on avoiding avalanches

check avalanche warning system
check local weather forecasts
avoid high risk terrain, ie. slopes of 30–45 degrees
avoid slopes with recent avalanche debris
beware of conditions where winds are above 20mph with snowfall
beware of rain and temperature rise after recent snowfall

Spring and autumn trekking is popular in the Himalayas and the number of walkers high climbing has quadrupled over the last decade. More than 10,000 people annually, trek across high passes round the Annapurna Massif. In this permanent winter terrain, the weather is usually stable, but in a mountain ecosystem violent changes can occur. Huge snowfalls and very wet snow cause avalanche and mudslides. Sixty-five trekkers and their supporters were engulfed and died in 1995 in one such unexpected storm.

Ski-injuries

Between 600,000 and 1,000,000 Britons take ski holidays abroad (Helal, 1992). The pastime attracts every age group, novices and experts, and is practised in a hostile terrain. Skiing is a potentially dangerous sport. The average overall injury rate is four per 1,000 skier days, with beginners experiencing approximately 60% of injuries and leg injuries accounting for 86%. According to the French Ski Resorts Doctors' Association there are about 110,000 winter ski accidents in the Alps every winter, a figure which has changed little in a decade despite many more skiers on the slopes. However, the number of serious ski accidents has increased alarmingly. Many hospitals in the Alps have reported a substantial increase in the number of patients who will never be able to walk again as a result of ski trauma. This trend is associated with faster skiing speeds, more skiers and the increasing popularity of dangerous, surf-style snow-boards.

In Switzerland for every 10,000 hours of sport, 13 ice hockey players, 10 footballers and 8 skiers have an accident and skiing is the third most dangerous sport in terms of accidental injury. Twelve percent of sports injuries result from ski trauma, which accounts for 30,000 incidents and 40% of those are serious. There are two accidents per 1000 skiers. An improvement in the statistics has been reported in the last few years due to improved boot bindings.

Sixty percent of knee injuries occur in women and 65% of shoulder injuries occur in men, probably due to a more aggressive style of skiing in males. Faster speeds increase the risk of injury to the upper body. Beginners are at higher risk with 13–18 casualties per 10,000m difference in altitude compared to good skiers with 3–5 casualties. Good skiers fall less frequently but have more serious injuries. Compression and centrifugal forces, which occur in modern downhill racing, exceed the endurance of the cartilage and tendo-ligament system. They cause overstrain injury in young racers.

Head injuries are more frequent when there is little snow on the piste.

Sites of ski injury recorded in 1991

45%	to knee
43%	tibial fractures
8%	to the arm
4%	to shoulder dislocation

The pattern of ski injury can vary from season to season and piste to piste. An Austrian doctor (Schlegel, 1997) responsible for a resort's trauma care, records:

Shoulder injuries	35%
Knee injuries	35%
Thumb injuries	8%
Tibia fractures	12%
Head injury	10%

Skiing competence and injury — casualties

58% were beginners
36% intermediate grade skiers
6% expert skiers

Recent years has seen an increase in the occurrence of knee injuries. Other accidents are due to collision with objects or other skiers. Injuries are caused by the use of drag-lines or chair-lifts and even the impact of bum-bags worn in front of the body. Fatigue can be an aggravating factor. Injuries are most likely to occur on the first day of the holiday and at the end of an afternoon session. Abrasions, lacerations, contusions and grazes to the knees are commonplace in skiers but the ski itself can cause other injuries. It acts as a lever on the leg, with relatively minor torque at the ski-lip causing a tibial fracture. Modern, rigid ski-boots minimise the risk of fracture but transfer stresses further up the leg to the knee, causing ligament damage round this joint.

Skis also cause lacerations and are dangerous projectiles if they come off and hurtle down the slope. Safety bindings react well to brief hard impacts but less well to gradually increasing rotational forces. One third of ski-induced injuries are serious. They often require surgery followed by intensive physiotherapy. The recovery period can be prolonged and may result in a substantial loss of income. **Precautionary measures** include for skiers include:

- ▶ correct adjustment of the ski binding
- ▶ training and development of leg muscles
- ▶ skiing within the skier's capabilities.

The condition known as '**skiing** thumb' is the result of falling on the outstretched hand with the thumb spread out. As this is a frequent type of accident, it is a wise practice to ski with the thumb outside the ski-pole hand loop. Ten percent of Alpine ski injuries are fracture of the ulnar collateral ligament of the thumb and the incidence has been estimated at 50–200,000 per annum (Peterson and Renstrom, 1992).

Ski-poles can cause abdominal perforations or eye injury and bum-bags have been known to cause trauma to the abdomen if they are worn at the front. If the pouch is full and hard, it can cause severe internal injury, such as a ruptured spleen or liver.

Ski-boot fracture of the lower leg is caused by failure of safety bindings to release the ski-boots during a fall. This injury causes greenstick fractures in children and is the most common injury suffered by skiers in their late teens. It is more likely to occur in powder snow conditions. Finger and thumb fractures are frequent on dry ski slopes when hands and fingers get jammed in the artificial fibre used for cladding the slopes.

Ski injuries can be serious. In ten recent ski accident victims, admitted to the National Spinal Injury Centre in Stoke Manderville Hospital, four had cervical spinal lesions. Downhill skiing fatalities are relatively infrequent with only 19 reported in the years 1980–90 in Alberta, Canada. The main causes of fatal accidents were travelling too fast, loss of control and collision (Tuff and Butt, 1993).

Caution should be observed near chairlifts as there is a danger that the unwary could be hit by moving machinery. Users of the chairlifts should always wait until the lift docks properly. Many accidents are caused to those who jump too soon and suffer trauma. T-bars and drag lifts are dangerous if misused and, as the lines are frequently out of sight of the operator, if an accident occurs, several skiers may be knocked over. T-bars can tangle in clothing and drag the skier up the slope. If care is not taken when undoing the T-bar it can rebound and injure other passengers.

Snow-boarding

Beginners at this sport are at greater risk than novice skiers, but injuries are usually less serious. Over 60% of all casualties are beginners in their first four days with men suffering 70% of snow-boarding injuries. The figures peak between 16 and 20 years of age. Fluctuations in age of holiday makers in different winter sports regions means that the percentage of snow-boarders on the slopes varies widely, but is increasing overall.

The division between 'Alpine' and 'free-style' boarding has led, not only to a difference in appearance and style performance, but also to the development of different boards, boots and injuries. As in skiing, injuries are distributed evenly between the upper and lower halves of the body. For 'Alpine' boarders, injuries to the leg are mainly to the knee joint, but for 'free-stylers' the softer boots increase the risk of injury to ankle joints. The main difference between skiing and snow-boarding, is in injuries to the wrist. Fracture of the radius bone at a typical point (fractura radii loco typico) is the most likely injury associated with this sport, accounting for between 31 and 41% of all snowboard injuries since 1991.

Ski and snow-board type of injury
>
> ski = knee
> snow-board = wrist

Prevention of snow-board injuries

Complicated jumps and landings put stress on the ankle and, increasingly, sports doctors are issuing warnings about damage to the upper and lower ankle. Support gloves should always be worn. Of 22 snow-boarders who broke their radius in the winter of 1996, only one was wearing support gloves.

Ice-skating

Ice-skating is popular and attracts skiers when the pistes are closed or there is a lack of snow. Contusions, lacerations and fractures from falls and collision with other skaters are frequent injuries, and skating on thin ice can cause death by drowning if the ice breaks. Novice skaters are more likely to suffer injury and should avoid overcrowded ice-rinks with poor crowd control.

Tobogganing/sledging

Experts use Olympic runs, but many resorts now cater for holidaymakers seeking the thrills of a more advanced track. Careless winter sports enthusiasts often slide down the slopes on improvised sledges and can suffer serious injury. The incidence of serious sledging accidents per annum is small, but the ratio to ski accidents is high (1:0.6) and, in relation to the length of holiday hours spent sledging, it is very high. Compared with motor cycling (a sport with very high risk of injury), there are disproportionate number of spinal injuries. In one report of 101 sledging accidents in eight days, there was one fatal head injury and five spinal injuries (Sloan and Matheson, 1985; Silver, 1993).

Hill climbing and mountaineering

In Europe, hills and mountains may be relatively safe in summer, but in winter when conditions are Arctic, they are much more dangerous. Travellers cross Europe to enjoy sporting holidays on Scottish mountains. Climbers regularly lose their lives in conditions which can be similar to those experienced in the Himalayas. Rescue teams record three main reasons for emergency call-out in Scotland and these are the same as those recorded by other European teams (Crockett, 1993):

1. Slips and falls when walking.

2. Being unable to proceed or retreat on a climbing route (crag-fast).

3. Entrapment and benightment on a hillside in poor weather conditions.

(McDonald, 1989)

In the Alps, avalanche and acute mountain sickness are added dangers. The most common injuries are to the head and lower leg, with hypothermia as an associated condition. In the year 1979–80, seven of the eight fatalities in Scotland were to unroped walkers or climbers (Liskiewicz, 1992), and a similar pattern occurs in Alpine and Himalayan mountain climbers. Difficult terrain means that rescue can be delayed and this compounds the effects of the injury.

As recreational use of Scottish mountains increases so, too, does the annual accident rate, and hypothermia was cited as a cause in 13% of all accidents occurring in the summer and winter of 1990. Accidental hypothermia is a common but sometimes undiagnosed condition in British hill climbing. Winter climbers are often ill-prepared for cold climatic extremes and fail to take into consideration the reduction in temperature associated with altitude.

Mishandling equipment, such as crampons or ice axes, can cause lacerations, abdominal perforation, rupture of internal organs and falls. Glissading, a common practice on steep snow fields, can become uncontrolled and the glissader can suffer similar traumata to sledgers. Uncontrolled glissaders can slide over cliffs.

Hill walkers

Most climbing accidents involve hill walkers and trekkers, rather than rock climbers. Falls on icy crags or snowslopes can cause fractures and internal injuries. Sprains, strains and contusions are frequent. Although minor, loss of mobility can trap the injured on a hillside after dark in poor weather conditions, increasing the risk of exposure and hypothermia.

High altitude climbers

Altitude sickness, hypoxia, hypothermia, over exposure to ultraviolet light and fluid loss are among the risks experienced by high altitude mountaineers. Fluid loss can amount to between 6 and 8 litres a day and is mainly from the respiratory tract. It is exacerbated by hypoxia-induced hyperventilation. The associated dehydration and haemoconcentration causes a rapid increase in blood viscosity which, in turn, reduces the oxygen-carrying capacity of the blood and tissue perfusion. Tissues deprived of oxygen readily succumb to frostbite and retinal haemorrhages and there is a risk of pulmonary and cerebral thrombosis (O'Donnell, 1979).

Ascent to over 3500m exposes individuals to the risk of hypoxia and physiological changes which can cause the following:

fluid retention
hyperventilation
respiratory alkalosis
pulmonary hypertension
increased blood viscosity
25% fall in cardiac stroke volume
25% increase in cerebral blood flow
erythropoetin secretion and polycythemia

Rapid ascent to high altitude exacerbates these changes so it is important to acclimatise the body, allowing it time to adjust.

Pre-travel counselling advice

Hypothermia

1.	Advise on the serious risks from hypothermia List signs and symptoms
2.	Recommend rainproof and windproof gear, woollen caps, gloves and jumpers
3.	Advise against wearing jeans which permit high heat loss from the lower half of the body
4.	Encourage winter sportsman to carry a survival bag
5.	Remind travellers of the dangers of wind-chill and wet clothing

Avalanche

If threatened, endeavour to ski and run to the side of the avalanche. If the individual is caught in an avalanch, arms should be flailed in a swimming motion to try to keep to the surface of the snow

Frostbite

Encourage the use of woollen gloves and balaclavas. Remind travellers of the signs of frostbite and of the need to warm the skin at the first sign of frostnip

Ultra-violet light

Advise travellers of the dangers of excess ultra-violet light radiation and of the intensity of UVL at high altitudes. The use of barrier creams and goggles or sunglasses should be recommended

Acute mountain sickness (AMS)

Remind travellers of the dangers of AMS when above 3,000m

Advise trekkers to only climb to recommended heights each day. Ideally, above 3000m, the net daily height gain should not exceed 500m

Recommend use of acetazoleamide as a prophylactic for AMS if climbing high

Advice to skiers

Ensure that bindings are correctly adjusted
Recommend the use of multi-mode release ski-bindings
Advise skiers to wear gloves and keep their thumbs out of ski-pole loops
Bum-bags should be worn on the back
Skiers should guard against fatigue from too much skiing, especially on the first day of their holiday

Advice to mountaineers

Remind mountaineers of the risks of hypothermia and exposure
List the symptoms of hypothermia
Suggest that they learn the correct use of an ice-axe for falls on snow and ice
Advise climbers to watch for weather change and loss of day-light

In winter climbing, careful preparation, sound route planning, weather-proof garments and boots, an eye to climatic change, avoidance of fatigue and the good sense to abort the expedition in bad climatic conditions is essential.

Additional advice for high altitude climbing and trekking

Restrict altitude gain to 500m per day over 3000m
Recommend the use of acetazolamide (Diamox) 500mg daily, taken 24 hours before proceeding over 4000m
Warn travellers of side-effects. A marked tingling of the arms and legs is common
Immediate return to a lower altitude is essential if there is evidence of high altitude pulmonary or cerebral oedema
Himalayan climbers can lose 6 to 8 litres of fluid per day and it is very important to maintain a very high water intake

Vaccinations

Sportsmen and women are at greater risk of trauma and infection than other travellers and they should be offered tetanus and hepatitis immunisation

Evacuation

The adverse effects of winter sports trauma can be compounded by delays in evacuation which may be measured in days rather than hours. In the higher peaks of the Himalayas and the Andes a week's walk may separate the climber from emergency aid. Helicopter rescue is unlikely and the only casualty transport is likely to be on a yak or Sherpa's back. Alpine and Scottish Highland Rescue Services use helicopters for rapid transportation out of the mountains but climatic conditions may make their use impracticable. Very expensive to operate, they may not be made available to the uninsured. Delays in finding the casualty and rescue team transportation by stretcher can be prolonged and hazardous. Delays in evacuation can kill hypothermic or badly traumatised sportsmen

Local medical facilities

Local medical facilities may be quite inadequate to meet the surgical and rewarming needs of the patient. The medical response in some countries may also not meet the criteria demanded of doctors in the UK.If there is trauma the need for surgery and transfusion arises. The patient may run the risk of transfusion with contaminated blood and has to consider the possibility of developing AIDS or hepatitis B. Lack of disposable instruments and equipment and poor sterilising and hygiene facilities may also bring infection risks from intervention procedures

Insurance

It is absolutely vital that winter sports enthusiasts have taken out adequate insurance.

A study in my own practice revealed a tendency for the young and perhaps the most at risk to avoid this extra financial outlay.

Even when insurance has been taken out, support is only as good as the proximity of the nearest rescue service, medical aid, the accessibility of the casualty and the climatic and environmental conditions which prevail

Sensible preparation

Simple precautions and an awareness of potential health dangers, a watch on the weather and state of day-light all help in minimising the risk for all involved in winter sports. Sound pre-travel counselling to winter sports enthusiasts may ensure that many of them come safely back from holiday

The provision of customised advice to the individual and provision of appropriate advice leaflets by health travel clinic personnel can help the travelling sportsman and woman to enjoy their sport abroad safely and return in good health

References

Crockett KV ed (1993) Scottish mountain accidents. *Scott Mountain Club J* **XXXV**(184): 308–12

Green M, Kerr A, McIntosh I, Prescott R (1981) Acetazolamide in the prophylaxis of acute mountain sickness. *Br Med J* **283**: 811–13

Helal P (1992) Skiing travellers health. In: Dawood R ed. *Travellers Health*. Oxford University Press, Oxford

Houston CS (1985) Incidence of AMS. *Am Alpine J* **27**: 161–2

Lehmuscallio E, Lindholm H, Koskenvuo K *et al* (1995) Frostbite of the face and ears. *Br Med J* 3111: 661–3

Liskiewicz WJ (1992) An evaluation of RAF S & R services in Britain. *J R Soc Med* **85**: 727–9

MacDonald CA (1989) Working with the team. *Scott Med J* **9**: 23–6

Maggiorini M, Buhler B, Walter M *et al* (1990) Prevalence of acute mountain sickness in the Swiss Alps. *Br Med J* **301**: 853–5

McIntosh IB (1986) Acetazolamide prophylaxis for AMS. *J Int Med Res* **14**(5): 285–7

McIntosh IB (1993) Man on the mountains — medical aspects. *Trav Med Int* **11**(4): 20–4

O'Donnell M (1979) We have ways of helping you climb the mountains. *World Med* **Jan 27**: 73

Peterson L, Renstrom P (1992) *Sports Injuries — Their Prevention and Treatment*. Martin Dunnitz, London

Pollard A (1992) Altitude-induced illness: If in doubt go down. *Br Med J* **304**: 1324–5

Roeggla G, Roeggla M, Binder M *et al* (1995) Effect of alcohol on body core temperature during cold weather immersion. *Br J Clin Pract* **49**: 239

Schlegel M (1997) Winter sports injuries in the Alps. *Scott Med J* **16**: 10–12

Silver JR (1993) The dangers of sledging. *Br Med J* **307**: 1602–3

Sloan JP, Matheson N (1985) How dangerous is sledging? *Br Med J* **290**: 821

Sneddon D (1993) Field management of hypothermic casualties arising from Scottish mountain accidents. *Scott Med J* **38**(4): 99–103

Tuff SC, Butt J (1993) Ski fatalities. *Am J Forensic Med Pathol* **14**: 12–16

Verbov J (1994) The sun and the skin. *Trav Med Int* **12**: 123–5

6

Health hazards and water sports

Watersports are a great attraction for holidaymakers abroad. Warm seas, shelving beaches, roaring surf, trade winds, racing rivers and winding waterways attract their own enthusiasts. Experts and novices sail, surf and canoe along shorelines and bays. The less adventurous, baked by the sun, plunge into swimming and rock pools, lochs, lakes and lagoons to cool off, ignorant of possible risks to health or the dangers of infection endemic at many of these destinations.

Each year avoidable deaths are reported, often due to drowning, hypothermia, diving injuries, boating and surfing accidents. Sports-induced infections can cause acute and chronic disease with prolonged morbidity. Local emergency medical and evacuation services may be excellent. However, in some popular international holiday resorts, especially those in developing countries, safety regulations are limited or absent, compliance poor and first aid training and medical facilities inadequate. In some cases treatment may add to the health risk because of poor hygiene and sterilisation, and contaminated equipment and blood products.

Pre-travel health advice from travel clinic staff should encourage holidaymakers to be more aware of these risks and the precautions that should be taken. Educational leaflets can be drawn up and given out. These are frequently available free of charge from local health authorities and pharmaceutical companies.

Swimmers

Rivers, lakes, lagoons and the open sea can be unpredictable. Foreign swimming pools, if neglected and not properly cleaned, should be avoided. They may be polluted or harbour bilharzia. The dangers of high diving into shallow pools should be stressed. A number of deaths from broken necks have occurred and even if the injured survive, permanent paralysis is a possibility (Grundy et al, 1991).

Men with an average age of 24 years are more likely to experience this injury and many have been drinking alcohol before they dive. A recent Scottish survey records this kind of injury as more common in Spain and Greece. The injury is often a crush fracture of a lower cervical vertebra, usually C5, with direct injury to the cord. Swimmers should avoid alcohol, look before they dive and not dive into less than 1.5m of water, or use a flat projectory dive.

Freshwater swimming away from the hotel has its own dangers. Popular coastal resorts may have sewage-polluted waters with the associated risk of conjunctivitis and ear infections. Swimming in the Mediterranean is more likely to cause gastrointestinal upsets (Dunlop, 1991) and algal bloom can contaminate freshwater lakes and estuaries. The blue-green algae (cyano bacteria) is toxic and swimmers should avoid contaminated water. Water contaminated with rat urine may cause leptospirosis. During the monsoon rains, rodents are flooded out of their nests on banks. This increases the risk of contaminating rivers with leptospires.

Leptospirosis in Thailand — case history

Two British travellers were on a raft expedition in Thailand when the raft capsized. They swallowed a considerable amount of water. A week later both were admitted to a Bangkok hospital after the abrupt onset of severe headache, myalgia and high fever. No diagnosis was made. They were discharged and later returned to Britain. Within days of their return, both were admitted to the infectious disease unit of a local hospital with aseptic meningitis caused by leptospirosis (Wolkans *et al*, 1988).

Schistomatosis

Many lakes and pools in Africa and the Middle East are infected with bilharzia (schistosomiasis) and tourists who swim in them can be infected.

The eggs of the intestinal worms hatch in water and infect certain kinds of snails. The larvae develop in the host and multiply, with some swimming free and penetrating the skin of a human host. In much of Africa, parts of the Middle East and Brazil the majority of the population is infected. Swimming or watersports in infected waters, especially where there are large areas of surface water, increases the risk of infection. Popular tourist spots in Africa such as Lakes Malawi, Victoria and Kariba are heavily polluted with schistosomes. 'Swimmers itch' is caused by schistosome larvae which have penetrated the skin and died there. They do not develop further but cause an intense itch, a form of cercarial dermatitis. It can occur in temperate as well as tropical countries and also in the USA. Fortunately, antihistamine tablets or ointment are all that is required for treatment.

Dracunculs medinensis (Guinea worm) is another source of infection in some popular tourist areas.

Deep waters, offshore cannot be considered safe. Lagoons can harbour *S. mansoni* and even small patches of water away from human habitation can be infected. Swimmers should never assume that fresh water is free from infection in an endemic area. Salt water, brackish water and chlorinated water are safe but neglected swimming pools can be colonised by the snails. Rubber boots and wetsuits offer protection for the watersportsman, but external clothing should be washed in uncontaminated water and dried quickly in the sun immediately after use. Artificial man-made lakes are particularly at risk of harbouring this infection.

Dangerous fish

Oceans and seas can present unexpected dangers for the unaware. Offshore winds, underground swells, thundering surf and treacherous currents should all be taken into account when swimming. There is also some risk of attacks by sharks, groupers, stingrays and crocodiles. Menstruating women may be apprehensive that menstrual blood will attract predators, but sharks and piranha are not attracted when blood is absorbed into sanitary towels or tampons. Aquatic leeches, prevalent in parts of South-east Asia, will gorge on any unprotected flesh. They will crawl into mouth, nostrils and eyes and swimming in forest pools and streams should be avoided.

Many fish and also sea anemones can inflict painful and dangerous stings. The coelenterates possess stings, especially on the tentacles. Contact results in severe burning pain followed by erythema and weals. With extensive stings from the Portuguese man-of-war, collapse may follow. Abrasions from corals can cause coral ulcers which take weeks to heal. Snorkellers and sailors in shallow waters should wear canvas shoes, which are some protection from abrasive coral but the sole can still be punctured by marine spines.

Hypothermia

Even in tropical waters, hypothermia can develop. If the water temperature is less than 21°C, protective suits should be worn. Without such protection, swimmers in water temperatures below 21°C this will lose heat faster than the body can renew it. Water conducts heat 25 times more rapidly than air and chilling and hypothermia can soon follow. At 5°C an unprotected swimmer will be in danger within 20 minutes of entering the water and will be dead within one hour and forty minutes. Temperature drops with increasing depth and the greatest change occurs after the first 10m, ie. below the range of penetration of the sun's warming effects.

Snorkelling

Brilliantly-hued fish are abundant in the bays and coral reefs of tropical seas. Snorkelling is a popular pastime but care should be taken if motor boats and jet skis are in the area. The snorkeller is often barely visible from above the water and these craft can inflict nasty injuries when travelling at speed. Use of goggles without a mouthpiece should be avoided because of the risk of bloodshot or black eyes. Trying to prolong the dive, by hyperventilating before starting to snorkel, is hazardous as it delays the build up of carbon dioxide. The snorkeller may use up all his/her oxygen and lose consciousness before the urge to surface and breathe again is felt. Hyperventilation before a dive has led to a number deaths from drowning.

Scuba-diving

The warm, clear waters of the Caribbean and Red Seas and the Pacific Ocean attract sub-aqua enthusiasts, and even experienced divers have failed to remember the dangers of nitrogen narcosis with deeper dives (Demberg, 1987). This is a physiological phenomenon of aqualung diving and not an irreversible pathological condition. When diving deeper than 16m with compressed air, the higher absolute partial pressures of nitrogen in the compressed air cause light-headedness, giddiness and impaired concentration. This disappears on returning to the surface. However, an intoxicated diver can act in a bizarre way when experiencing the 'Rapture of the Deep', disregarding safe diving principles and ignoring safe ascent procedures. Decompression sickness can quickly follow (Stewart, 1989).

Nitrogen dissolved in the tissues must be allowed to remain in solution in the blood stream and eventually exhaled. Decompression sickness is caused by the formation and circulation of bubbles of nitrogen gas which come out of solution and body tissues during ascent. These bubbles form if the diver is submerged for a relatively long time or comes up too fast. They can occlude small arteries and veins and cause physiological dysfunction in joints and bones, the central nervous system and the lungs. Abdominal cramps, dehydration, diarrhoea and fever are contraindications to safe diving. If a diver is suffering from a gastrointestinal upset it is dangerous to dive.

Scuba divers risk decompression sickness if they fly home immediately after a dive. Aircraft cabin pressure can create enough of a pressure gradient between the lower cabin ambient pressure and higher tissue pressures of nitrogen remaining from the dive, to cause some bubble formation and subsequent decompression sickness. No dive greater than 9m should be taken within 24 hours of a flight and, even after shallow no-decompression dives, at least 12 hours should elapse before flying (Ridout, 1992).

Easy access to scuba facilities attracts novices to the sport. Equipment in developing countries may be less than reliable and compressed air supplies can be of variable quality. Instructions on diving safety are often much below the standard of those in Britain and novice divers may be encouraged to dive without adequate training and supervision. They may be taught by poorly qualified instructors and language constraints make communication difficult. Diving operators are often looking for quick financial returns and tutorials may consist of a short, superficial programme and inadequate instruction. Inadequate teaching in the early stage can be hazardous and novices risk barotrauma even when practising in deeper swimming pools.

If novice aqualung divers hold their breath during rapid ascent from depth, pulmonary problems, such as air embolism, pneumothorax and mediastinal emphysema, may develop. Expanding air inside the lungs may rupture the alveoli with tracking of the air into the pulmonary venous system and interstitial tissues. Women divers with significant pre-menstrual symptoms should not dive as severe cramps can affect concentration and mimic the signs of decompression sickness (McIntosh, 1991). Pregnant women are advised not to dive at all as little is known of deep diving effects on the developing foetus.

Divers who are asthmatic should not dive for 48 hours after a wheezy attack (Farrel and Glanville, 1990). Even if only mildly wheezy, there is a risk that sections of lung might be incompletely ventilated as the diver ascends. These sections may fail to empty sufficiently resulting in pneumothorax or gas embolism (Douglas, 1983).

AIDS

The UK Health and Safety Executive publication 'AIDS, HIV infection and Diving' confirms that HIV cannot be transmitted by breathing apparatus or during first-aid procedures taught to divers (Health and Safety Executive, 1991).

Surfing and boating

The sight of experienced surfers, hotdogging across the face of a 10 foot curl on a breaking wave attracts many to this sport. Injuries to novices are especially frequent, and are usually the result of being struck by their own or another's board. Abrasions and gravel burns are common. Body surfers are at highest risk of sustaining severe injuries (Harries, 1980). These are sustained when waves are steep and break precipitously; the wave is known as a 'dumper' and it rams the surfer headfirst into the sea-bed. The neck is forcefully flexed and rotated, causing fractures to the skull and cervical spine. The head also can hit a hidden sandbank in steep dives in shallow water, causing major fracture and, possibly, tetraplegia.

Windsurfing is another popular pastime Dangers include collapsing booms, falling masts and capsize. In falls from surfboards in shallow lagoons, feet can be impaled on sea urchins' spines, which are capable of penetrating plastic beach shoes. Lightly clad sportsmen may suffer hypothermia, fatigue and exhaustion if their board is swept out to sea. Novice windsurfers should always sail into the wind and along the shores. Offshores winds are prevalent off many islands, blowing the unwary out to sea. Inexperienced surfers may find it impossible to return to shore. Rescue boats may be unmanned, unserviceable or payment may be required in advance. Rescue may depend on chance on-shore observation. The quality of service may be inadequate in the event of an emergency. Small boat hirers may be more interested in saving their boat rather than the life of the hirer.

Water-skiing

Water-skiing off crowded holiday beaches carries the risk of collision with other skiers and swimmers. Skiers may find that local waters are contaminated with algae. Inhaling or swallowing algal bloom, present in fresh, esturine and marine waters can cause pneumonia (Philipp,

1992). Women water-skiers are at risk of ascending vaginal infections and should wear swimwear that protects the perineum adequately.

Barefoot water skiing has its enthusiasts and requires both skill and courage. With the tow boat travelling at speeds in excess of 45mph there are real risks of spinal cord injury. Water hitting the perineum at high speed can also cause trauma. Sudden failure of wet-suit stitching can result in high speed rectal and vaginal douching and rectal and vaginal tears and salpingitis may follow.

Case history

> An orthopoedic surgeon recorded massive muscle breakdown from a high speed barrage of water he experienced when learning barefoot water skiing. He developed haematuria and myoglobinuria (Barrat, 1990).

Adequate protection, such as wet or dry suits must be worn. A high wind chill factor when being towed at speed is typical even in tropical resorts.

Small boat sailing

Sailing and rowing boats, pedalos, canoes and jet skis are favoured by novices and the experts at many resorts. Collisions or blows from swinging booms that may cause trauma and falls into fast currents and tidal races, which may sweep the injured away. These are some of the hazards that need to be considered. Holidaymakers, who capsize into algae-covered waters, may develop pneumonia or, if waters are rat-infested, leptospirosis. Organisms of the *Leptospira interrogans* complex can enter the body through a skin cut or abrasion or, more commonly, through the intestinal tract. Drowning, hypothermia and exposure are risks associated with all water sports, and caution and safety awareness should be practised.

On-shore water enthusiasts

Tourists wandering along the shore line or paddling in the shallows are less at risk from trauma but are still at risk from infection by larva migrans. The hookworm larva infects the sand above the water mark. Discarded from the intestine of dogs and cats, it burrows into and penetrates human skin, causing itchy, red lines (Verbov, 1989). Larval infection is common on Caribbean beaches and can usually be avoided if beach shoes are used.

Sandflies and mosquitoes may also plague shorelines. Skin should be covered to reduce the risk of bites from these insects, which often cause localised or systemic infection. It is sensible to apply insect repellants before being bitten.

Reflected light and exposure to the sun can cause severe sun burn. Fair skinned Europeans on short, sea resort holidays are most likely to suffer. Their obsession with acquiring a tan in spite of the risk of over-exposure which may ruin their holiday, can be a major cause of skin cancer in the young and increase the risk of onset of cerebrovascular ischaemia and stroke in older age groups. Tourists should be reminded that actinic rays pass through thin materials and water and cause severe burns, dehydration and febrile illness. High factor sun screens (at least sun protection factor 25 (25SPF)) which are water-resistant should be applied and reapplied during exposure to intense sunlight.

Parasailing instructions for takeoff from the beach or water are often minimal. Tourists may not speak the local language and trainers may not speak English so communication can be difficult. Take off from land and water may be risky and depend on the skills of the towing boatman. Fractures can occur as most parasailers are making their first, uninitiated landing. In some resorts the return is hampered by a steep descent over tall apartments, busy streets and a tree-lined beach. The parasailor may be buffeted by capricious winds and have little time to prepare for landing. Safety depends on a tow rope of questionable reliability and boatmen who are motivated more by financial considerations than safety.

Bungee jumping off bridges and tower cranes into or just above the water is now an established vacational exploit. Cheered on by the more sensible and safety conscious, the young and not so young throw themselves into the air, tied to an elastic line to restrain their headlong downward plunge. At popular sites, teams of people dive at minute intervals. Jumpers are clipped on to ropes that may be inadequate or unreliable and would be rejected by reputable mountaineers. Bungee jumping takes place over rivers used by canoes and jet boats. There is no communication between jumpers and their instructors and, in some instances, they have collided with the people in boats.

There has been a substantial increase in the number of injuries to the eyes and face of participants in this sport. These injuries include contusions and haemorrhages of the eyes and facial structure, possibly caused by the quick changes in air pressure occuring during the jumps. The sudden increase in air pressure can cause ruptures of the small capillaries which supply blood to the retina (Krott, 1997).

Although the young may survive relatively unscathed, older people are at risk of disc injuries and fractures. Bouncing up and down on the end of the rope after the fall increases the risk of cardiac and cerebrovascular accident. Yet 50- and 60-year-olds are frequent participants.

The majority of jumpers bounce above the water at the end of the rope. Some choose to 'wet bungee', ie. where the elastic tether is long enough to immerse the jumper in the water. When these enthusiasts hit the water they can sustain injury from high velocity impact pressures. This impact can cause retinal haemorrhage and even facial fracture.

Case history

> *A man completed a 160 foot bungee dive into a river, felt pain in his right eye and noticed blood coming from his nostril. He had haemorrhaging in both eye lids and in the right retina and was thought to have a fractured facial bone (Krott, 1997).*

People who bungee jump are seldom aware of the health risk they run. Those who participate are often on tour. The medical accidents suffered are reported to different centres across the world and are poorly collated. Elderly people should be firmly persuaded against taking part and health professionals should advise young and old of the injuries that are caused by this very dangerous sport.

Ship-to-shore transfer

Although few elderly people are water sports enthusiasts, an increasing number are exposed to the risks of small boat transport in ship-to-shore transfers (see *Chapter 4, Page 33–35*).

Doctors and nurses at the travel health clinic or general practice surgery should make sure that the frail and those with mobility problems are advised about these problems. If tender transfers are part of the cruise, elderly people concerned about safety should be advised to stay onboard and forego the excursions. Local medical facilities vary in quality in foreign ports and if fractures or dislocations are sustained, treatment may be inadequate.

Safety

Safety consciousness is not a priority in many foreign holiday resorts and few water-sportsmen or women and travellers are aware of the inadequacy of local medical facilities. Good emergency care and evacuation at many destinations may be limited or unavailable, a situation not appreciated by vacationers until they need such a service.

> Despite a catalogue of possible disasters, the majority of tourists travel and enjoy their water activities free from harm. By remaining alert to potential risks, taking sensible safety precautions, and appreciating and respecting the possible risks associated with local conditions, most holidaymakers can safely enjoy their sport.

Travel health clinic advice

Health professionals in travel health clinics should be prepared to counsel sports enthusiasts on the risks associated with watersports. Travel vaccination consultations provide the opportunity and advice can be reinforced with information leaflets. It should be stressed that facilities for treating trauma abroad may be inadequate and healthcare poor. There is also risk of contracting HIV and hepatitis infections. These may be caused by the use of contaminated blood products or instruments and this should be mentioned.

Leaflet advice

Water and beach sports

- ► check all equipment personally before use
- ► ensure that safety precautions and regulations exist and are complied with
- ► obtain adequate instruction in the chosen sport, in English if possible or with a good translator
- ► check the availability of good first aid and emergency medical treatment

- assess the quality of local medical facilities, ie. hospitals, clinics and equipment
- make sure that insurance protection covers the sport.

Water sports

- wear protective shoes on beaches and in small craft
- wear a bouyancy aid
- avoid water where bilharzia is prevalent
- avoid still waters contaminated with algal bloom
- use insect repellent
- wear high protection factor sun screeen
- be extra cautious when sailing with offshore winds
- do not drink before diving
- check the depth of the pool before diving
- use flat trajectory dives and only dive into water more than 1.5 metres deep

Subaqua divers

- use reputable companies who comply with internationally recognised scuba-diving regulations
- use qualified instructors with a good command of English or good translation facilities
- ensure introductory courses are of regulation duration and content
- check the equipment personally
- adhere to the rules for safe diving
- do not hold the breath when ascending
- asthmatic divers should not dive within 48 hours of an attack
- do not dive deeper than 9 metres within 24 hours of a flight
- do not dive at all within 12 hours of a flight.

References

Barrat DS (1990) Can orthopoedic surgeons walk on water. *Br Med J* **301**:1429–30

Demberg M (1987) Health advice for travelling scuba divers *Trav Med Int* **6**: 61–5

Douglas DM (1983) Shallow water air diving. *Scott Med J* **1**:18–19

Dunlop J (1991) Blooming algae. *Br Med J* **302**: 671–2

Farrell S, Glanville P (1990) Diving practices of scuba drivers with asthma. *Br Med J* **300**: 166

Grundy D, Penney P, Graham L (1991) Diving into the unknown. *Br Med J* **302**: 670–1

Harries MG (1980) Surfing and surfing injuries. *Medisport* **2**: 106–7

Health and Safety Executive (1991) IND(G)101L. Health and Safety Executive, London

Krott R (1997) Orbital emphysema as a complication of bungee jumping. *Med Sci Sports Exercise* **29**: 850–2

McIntosh IB (1991) The health of the woman traveller. *Trav Med Int* **9**: 24–8

Philipp R (1992) Algal Blooms. In: Dawood R, ed. *Travellers' Health*. Oxford University Press, Oxford

Ridout S (1992) Water and water sports. In: Dawood R, ed. *Travellers' Health*. Oxford University Press, Oxford

Stewart K (1989) The rapture of the deep. *Scott Med J* **7**: 8–10

Verbov J (1989) Skin hazards of travel. *Trav Med Int* **7** 143–7

Wolkans E, Cope A, Watkins S (1988) Rapids, rafts and rats. *Lancet* **21**: 283–4

7

Healthcare of the expeditioner, backpacker and adventurer

Residents in the UK visited six million destinations outside Europe in 1992 (Business Monitor, 1992). The majority toured popular routes in Africa, Asia and the Far East and usually travelled on package holidays protected from contact with local people. Most travellers have been vaccinated, are compliant with malaria prophylaxis, stay in deluxe hotels and have good insurance protection. Some suffer from sunburn, too much food and alcohol, insect bites and travellers' diarrhoea, but the majority return home without any major ill effects.

More adventurous travellers ignore mass market holidays and draw up their own itinerary to remote areas of the world. They climb inaccessible mountains, cross arid deserts and explore rainforests and Arctic wastes. Such travellers are exposed to extremes of temperature (Melville, 1984), high altitude (Illingworth, 1984), hostile terrain, exotic disease, psychological stress and physical trauma. Although the majority take personal health precautions, some ignore the possible risks to well-being.

Health risks

Other groups who suffer similar health risks include young world travellers, those travelling without sufficient money and backpackers (Reid and Cossar, 1994). They stay with local families, eating local cuisine which may carry infections to which tourists are more susceptible than local people. They frequently live in cheap and squalid accomodation with unhygienic toilet provision, exposed to animal- and insect-transmitted diseases and exotic infections.

Campers are at risk from climate changes, rugged terrain and, especially, vector-borne disease. Personal health provision for foreign travel is often inadequate. They may not be vaccinated against common diseases endemic in the country in which they are travelling and refuse prophylaxis and antimalarial medication. Although many travel without ill-effects, others acquire infections, such as HIV, hepatitis, malaria and tropical disease, or suffer physical trauma. Few fully appreciate the inherent health risks of vacation activities.

Sea-sickness, saltwater sores, sunburn, exposure and hypo-thermia can affect travellers on boat, raft or canoe expeditions and decompression sickness is a risk if diving regulations are ignored (see *Chapter 6*). Dehydration affects travellers at high altitudes or in dry terrain, and acute mountain sickness (AMS) is a risk for those travelling above 3000m (see *Chapter 5*), as is hypothermia, frostbite and ultraviolet radiation. Expeditioners through jungles and rainforests can suffer heat exhaustion, trench foot and insect and leech bites.

Expeditioners and adventurers seeking advice from doctors and travel agents are often poorly advised. Advice is not specific enough to the destination and planned itinerary (Mott and Kinnersley, 1990; Gorman, 1992). Medical care for this type of travel should consist of more than advice on the contents of a first-aid kit. General practice travel health clinics can meet these needs by identifying possible risks, conducting a clinical examination if necessary, organising appropriate vaccination and advocating sensible precautions.

Physical injury

The risk of physical trauma is high on adventure holidays (McIntosh, 1993b). Sprains, strains, contusions and fractures are a possiblility and a first-aid kit is essential. Expedition groups may have access to extensive first-aid chests, but solo back-packers often grudge the extra weight of a few pills and plasters.

Table 7.1: Contents of a first-aid kit for the adventure traveller (continued)

- paracetamol/ibuprofen/aspirin
- bandages, adhesive tape, gauze/wound dressings, tube gauze
- scissors, safety pins, tweezers
- anti-diarrhoeal tablets, eg. Loperamide
- oral rehydration preparation, eg. Diarolyte
- sunscreen (high protection factor, eg. x25)
- antihistamine (cream and tablets)
- water purification tablets and equipment
- dental kit

Table 7.1: Contents of a first-aid kit for the adventure traveller

- insect repellent containing 'Deet'
- motion sickness medications, eg. Hyoscintabs
- thermometer
- antimalarial drugs (stand-by and prophylactic); broad spectrum antibiotics (for travel to remote areas)
- anti-AIDS kit (needles, syringes, sutures, IV cannula, sterilising swabs)
- condoms/contraceptive pills
- tampons and toilet paper
- antiseptic preparations
- topical antibiotic/antifungal ointments

Simple trauma is the most common presenting feature on most expeditions. Lacerations, abrasions, contusions and blisters are commonplace. Ignored or inadequately treated, they can become infected and threaten the success of the expedition. Insect and leech bites can cause infection and may need antibiotic treatment.

Case history

An expeditioner on a walking trip in Central American jungle, developed a simple paronychia from a tiny skin tear at the side of one nail. It was a minor wound and not painful. He decided to lance it himself and did so with an unsterilised safety pin. It quickly became infected and abscessed into a painful and throbbing wound. The expedition doctor treated it with penicillin which had no effect. In a few days the patient had lymhadenitis stretching up the arm and had become febrile.

A high dose of second antibiotic showed no benefit and he became very ill, unfit to proceed and held up progress of the party. The first-aid kit carried no other medication. His evacuation was essential and team members had to carry him out of the jungle and organise his transfer to hospital. This took several days. In the hospital the bacteria in the wound and in his blood stream was quickly identified and an appropriate antibiotic was given. He recovered but the expedition had to be abandoned. Two years preparation and fundraising had come to nothing due to a very minor wound.

Road traffic accidents

Road traffic accidents are the major cause of trauma in developing countries (*see Chapter 2*) and are a particularly common cause of fatalities in travellers in their teens and early twenties. Airlines in developing countries have poor safety records and road transport is frequently mechanically unsound, overloaded, lacks seatbelts, and is driven by drivers with limited skills who are inebriated or on drugs. Roads are inadequately maintained, ill-lit, narrow and congested.

Travellers hire scooters, cars and motor-cycles and do not check to make sure that these are roadworthy or whether the brakes work. They drive off without protective clothing or helmets. They also ride horses, camels, mules and yaks over vertiginous trails and high altitude passes, and can suffer falls, abrasions, fractures and bites.

Simple first-aid care is usually all that is necessary, but at high altitude or in the tropics, even small wounds can become infected.

Water transport and trauma

Water transport lacking basic safety equipment is often used by travellers to remote areas. There is a high risk of boats capsizing, causing hypothermia and drowning. Accidents are common when running river rapids in inflatable craft. Stopper waves can cause an abrupt change of course and striking rocks and cliffs can result in serious injury.

Pre-travel consultations should identify possible forms of transport and draw attention to potential risks of physical trauma or infection. Protective helmets and lifejackets are usually unobtainable in developing countries and, if feasible, should be carried from the UK. If crossing potentially infected waters cannot be avoided, sensible precautions would be to cross upstream of villages and to wear boots and clothing in the water.

Expeditioners may be bitten by insects and are at risk of infections from mosquitoes, blackflies, and sandflies. Malaria, dengue fever and Japanese encephalitis can be caused by unprotected exposure. 'Travellers rests' often have fleas and bed-bugs and, when walking the trails, there is the risk of leech bites or meeting rabid dogs and monkeys. Adequate primary medical care is unlikely to be available locally and the quantity and quality of any local facilities or professional skills may be well below optimal standards of care.

Backpackers and expeditioners are constrained by the amount of gear that can be carried and will usually only take the minimum necessary for survival. This should include mosquito nets, insect repellents, water sterilising equipment, a first-aid kit and an anti-AIDS kit. If the travel clinic does not supply these kits, it should have lightweight samples available and on display. Encouraging a sensible, attitude to safety and lifestyle abroad is vital and may prevent morbidity or even fatality.

Precautions highlighted by the clinic should include water sterilisation, avoidance of suspect foods and scrupulous attention to hand-washing and personal hygiene in food preparation in camps along the trail.

Infections

Backpacking and expeditioning often includes visits to regions where malaria, hepatitis and HIV infection are common (see *Chapter 8*). Close association with the local population increases the risks of catching infective disease. Package travellers in a tour group are more likely to be shielded from such infection (Walker, 1994). If malaria is endemic, malaria prophylaxis and compliance is essential. Medication does not offer complete protection, but use of repellants, mosquito nets and adequate cover-up clothing reduces the risk of bites.

Gastroenteritis

If the quality of living accommdation is poor, travellers are more likely to suffer gastrointestinal (GI) disease. When comparing travellers staying in a deluxe hotel with others living more simply in less salubrious accommodation, studies show that there is a marked difference in the number of people seeking medical attention (Chatterjee, 1993). The hotel residents have a lower incidence of GI illness and the adventurers are more likely to be affected to varying degrees. Some illnesses are only a nuisance, settling within a few days. Others are much worse and people may be affected by *E.coli*, *Salmonella*, *Shigella*, *Giardia* organisms, parasites and rotaviruses, and return home with the illness (Okhuysen, 1992). Campers and backpackers usually live rough, near rural villages in close proximity to local people. They are at high risk of contracting diarrhoea and vomiting. Travellers' diarrhoea is the single most common problem affecting travellers and bacterial infections account for up to 80% of cases (Walker, 1994).

Organisms causing diarrhoea

Organism	%
E.coli	40
Shigella	15
Salmonellas	10
Rotaviruses	10
Giardia lamblia	3
E.histolytica	3
Enteropathogens (cholera; typhoid)	19

Nutrition

All water should be considered contaminated and treated by boiling, chemical sterilisation and/or filtering. Food is likely to be contaminated if bought locally and should be cooked, boiled or peeled. On commercial expeditions to the Himalayas and Africa, food is often prepared by local cooks and guides. Scarcity of water and poor hygiene standards increase the risk of food being infected and causing gastrointestinal upset. Infection can be caused by food, fluids, unwashed hands, filth, flies, drinking and eating utensils. Information leaflets should be available in the travel health clinic and the GP surgery. These can reinforce advice on prevention.

AIDS

Many developing countries have a higher prevalence of human immunodeficiency virus (HIV) than the UK. Travellers should be reminded that 80% of all cases of acquired immunodeficiency syndrome (AIDS), registered in Britain and contracted heterosexually, were acquired abroad (Reid and Cossar, 1994).

Counsellors should advise travellers of the dangers of unprotected sex. If sexual abstinence is not observed, condoms should be carried by individual travellers. Women should be reminded that they are two to four times more at risk than men, of contracting AIDS from unprotected intercourse.

Lyme borreliosis

Lyme borreliosis is a tick-borne disease caused by *spirochaetes* and occurs throughout the northern hemisphere with high endemicity in parts of the United States and Sweden. Hikers and trekkers can be infected from deer ticks. The risk of infection can be reduced by simple practical precautions such as tucking socks into boots, wearing boots and long trousers and inspecting skin and clothing for ticks.

Sunlight

Excessive exposure to sunlight causes premature skin ageing, and increases the risk of skin cancer and cataracts. Effects from the sun can be aggravated by reflection from water, snow and sand, high altitude, drugs and extreme latitudes.

Travellers should carry ultraviolet screens with sun protective factor of 15 plus. The hole in the ozone layer makes exposure to sunlight particularly dangerous for lake and offshore sailors in the southern latitudes of Chile and Argentina. Due to the rarified atmosphere, climbers in the high Andes are at risk, not only from ultraviolet rays, but also during travel over high snowfields and glaciers. These have high light reflection and can cause severe sunburn and snow blindness if sunscreen creams and goggles are not used.

High altitude climbers and expeditioners run additional risks from exposure to cold, acute mountain sickness, hypothermia and dehydration. Climbers must keep their fluid input high.

Acute mountain sickness (AMS)

Travellers above 3000m are at risk of AMS and should be made aware of the dangers of this condition (see *Chapter 5*). It can be fatal. Prophylactic use of acetazolamide is recommended at a dose of one 250mg tablet per day, taken 24 hours in advance of exposure to over 3000m altitude. Susceptibility to this disease cannot be predicted, although the young, who may travel too high, too fast and too far each day, appear at highest risk. As soon as symptoms present, all high altitude travellers should either rest at that level, or return to a lower level (Green *et al*, 1981; McIntosh and Prescott, 1986).

Dehydration

Dehydration is a risk for those crossing dryer and higher areas. The first few days in very hot zones are potentially the most dangerous. An unacclimatised person will secrete only half the volume of sweat he/she secretes when acclimatised ten days later. There is a high risk of heat stroke if initial body heat regulation is poor.

Any person suffering febrile illness or from conditions which cause loss of fluid, such as gastroenteritis are at risk of heat disorder. After sunset, at low altitudes, temperatures in the Sahara can fall below freezing and wind chill effects can be substantial in deserts. Travellers can suffer from cold exposure despite being overheated all day (Lewis, 1965; Barber, 1978).

Expeditions over water

The great rivers of the world attract the expeditioner and today's explorers set off across the oceans and large lakes, challenging previous feats of endurance. Groups sail, canoe and raft across wide expanses of water in remote areas. Lacerations, haematomata, abrasions, rope burns, galley scalds and blisters from oars and paddles are commonplace. These are easily infected and often slow to heal. Sea sickness can be disabling until the individual becomes accustomed to the rolling movement caused by waves (Illingworth, 1984). Other problems that can affect these travellers are dehydration, salt depletion (Leech, 1978), illness caused by heat and, in icy seas, hypothermia.

On stormy seas and large inland lakes, waves can be many feet high and may capsize the boat or sweep the unwary overboard. Unless survival techiques are put into action, fatalities can result (Forrester, 1987). Feet exposed to water temperatures just above freezing for long periods can be affected by trenchfoot, a disorder which causes immersion injury. Symptoms are loss of sensation and damage to skin and muscles. Sea water sores are also common.

Repetitive movements to tendons during canoeing and rowing can cause tenosynovitis, crippling arms and wrists. Capsize is common in white water canoeing and rafting, and there is a high risk of fractures and skull injury if the craft hits rocks. Commercial rafting on many foreign rivers is done without helmets and scant attention is given to safety precautions (McIntosh, 1991). Sudden immersion in waters contaminated with *Schistomatosis*, *Leptospirosis*, guinea worm and cyanobacteria can cause infection (Philip, 1992; Hardy, 1998).

Emergency evacuation

In some instances, evacuation may mean being carried on a Sherpa's back, or prolonged travel on unmade roads in unsprung vehicles. Insurance cover, if purchased, is useless if the nearest care unit is too distant to be reached. Physical trauma and casualty care in many parts of the world carry the risk of HIV infection from infected blood products and contaminated needles. Many insurance companies meet this challenge by rapidly evacuating the injured person to a hospital centre where blood samples are untainted. However, the unconscious, haemorrhaging or dehydrated patient may need immediate care to survive. Transfusion supplies available locally may be used, and may carry the risk of HIV infection.

Expedition groups may carry sterile packs, needles, intravenous drip sets and infusion material to avoid this risk, but the additional weight of such kits is a deterrent to the backpacker and high climber. Travel health professionals should emphasise these dangers to such travellers.

Hospitalisation

Emergency units and hospitals may be many miles from the scene of an accident. Even when accessible, resources are often limited and buildings and equipment antiquated. In Bhutan, wards are unheated and hold many tuberculous patients. In India and Pakistan, they are grossly overcrowded and meals may only appear if supplied by relatives. Hospitals in Nepal and Kashmir may have stone slabbed floors and beds jammed together, with unsuitable, unhygienic toilet facilities. In eastern Europe and Russia, payment to the nursing orderly may be required before personal attention for toileting will be provided.

Treatment in rural areas of China often depends upon acupuncture and herbal medicine. These areas may lack even the simplest medical equipment. In large areas of Asia and Africa disposable equipment is unavailable, sterilisation of reusable rubber and glass items unpredictable and water supplies suspect or rationed.

Injured and ill adventurers are usually given the best treatment available, but that may be well below the standard of hospitals in Western Europe or the United States. Trekkers and high climbers should be reminded that accident and insurance protection cover is only as good as the quality of the nearest emergency unit and its staff.

Post travel illness

Some travellers return home with travel-acquired illness. In a study of trekkers visiting Nepal, India and Morocco, half were ill during the trek, and usually affected by diarrhoea. The illness experienced in Morocco was of such severity that 40% of clients had to miss part of the trek itinerary. One third of all trekkers reported continuing illness, usually gastrointestinal, in the month after returning home. Diarrhoea was the usual symptom. Those visiting Nepal were most likely to consult the family doctor on their return (Townend, 1998).

The travel health clinic

The majority of those travelling abroad return home without suffering major ill health. Counselling in pre-health travel consultations can help to further reduce traveller morbidity. Health professionals should identify high-risk travellers who need specific advice from the travel clinic, health centre or general practitioner. The travel health clinic has an obligation to educate this group of travellers about the health risks that they are likely to meet, and should carry out a personalised health assessment. This needs to be based on destination, objectives, routes, methods of travel, season and local endemic disease.

Management programme

A management programme tailored to the traveller should include appropriate prophylaxis, which depends on a realistic appraisal of the likely disease exposure. Only around five per cent of travel-related diseases are vaccine-preventable.

The travel health clinic consultant should allocate sufficient time to provide advice on how to avoid potential health problems and to discussing vaccination procedures. Staff should also draw the traveller's attention to his/her personal responsibility for maintaining good health when abroad. This may require modification of behaviour and lifestyle (McIntosh, 1993a).

Information and advice can be reinforced by providing appropriate leaflets. These should cover:

► water sterilisation
► food hygiene

▶ insect-borne disease, infections

▶ high altitude effects

▶ adverse effects of ultraviolet light and mortality.

Vaccination and prophylaxis are only part of health protection. Consideration should also be given to destination, routes, transport methods and daily living during the time abroad. The initial consultation should identify potential hazards. These can be drawn to the traveller's attention and appropriate pre-travel preparation advised. High-risk travellers, although a minority group, require individual assessment and counselling to ensure that their journey achieves maximum benefits and they return in good health. Assessment of risk depends on:

▶ current health status and medications

▶ previous history of cardiac disease

▶ previous history of respiratory disease

▶ history of travel sickness

▶ history of acute mountain sickness

▶ history of asthma, diabetes and allergies

▶ physical examination if indicated

▶ provision of immunisation and prophylaxis

▶ recommendations on an appropriate first-aid kit

▶ consideration of specific risks associated with the expedition.

Case history A

On a badly organised trip to Kilimanjaro, a man joined the group at the last moment. He was not well known to the others but they needed the extra finance that he brought to expedition funds. When climbing on Mount Kilimanjaro, he became dehydrated and collapsed, semiconscious and uncommunicative. The attempt to reach the top had to be abandoned. His survival was in doubt. It was then discovered that he was a non-insulin dependent diabetic. His fluid and food intake were impaired as he climbed and the extra exertion and effects of altitude had caused metabolic imbalance. Fortunately a doctor on another expedition was able to resuscitate him. He ruined the climbing venture for the rest of his team and nearly died in his attempt to reach the summit.

Case history B

A senior expeditioner came close to medical disaster at the very beginning of one adventure trip when time was at a premium and lost days could ruin the expedition's chances of success. Allergic to lobster, he inadvertently ate crustaceans in a sea food platter at a wayside eating place, just before the team's flight into remote jungle. He became unconscious with breathing compromised. Following cardiopulmonary resuscitation he recovered but was debilitated by diarrhoea and vomiting. As he was leading the expedition, the viability of whole project was threatened. Fortunately, with medication from a comprehensive medical emergency kit, his recovery was rapid and the group had a successful venture.

Case history C

A key climber on one trip jeopardised his party when he failed to reveal that he was on drug therapy. Suffering from a dental abscess, he had been prescribed metronidazole. He did not recall any specific instructions about the avoidance of alcohol and had a complimentary drink on the aeroplane taking the group to a small air strip. This lay at the base of the mountain they were to climb.

He suddenly felt ill and became unconscious. On a small aeroplane, emergency aid was unavailable and laying him in a prostrate position was impracticable. There appeared no cause for the sudden collapse and only the simplest life support measures could be practised. The closest landing airfield had few emergency facilites and good medical aid was many miles away.

The climber had suffered a violent drug interaction. Metronidazole has a disulfiram-like reaction with alcohol. On landing he recovered consciousness. Careful history taking revealed the cause of the collapse and he was fit enough to climb in 24 hours. As the skilled lead mountaineer, he had nearly jeopardised success for the other climbers and put his own life at risk.

Immunisations

A comprehensive immunisation programme, tailored to specific health risks is required for these expedition travellers. Unfortunately, because they are travelling on a tight budget, the people most likely to benefit from prophylactic immunisation are not always prepared to pay the medical costs.

Typhoid, yellow fever, tetanus, polio, hepatitis A and B, rabies, and tuberculosis immunisation should be considered if travelling for over a month through rural areas in Asia, or if going on extended backpacking trips through Africa, Nepal and Northern India. Some adventurers will require Japanese encephalitis and meningitis protection. Tick-borne encephalitis occurs in forested regions in Europe and Scandinavia. This protection should be offered to walkers and campers visiting these areas between June and September.

Malaria

Adventure travellers are at high risk from insect bite infection. Malaria prophylaxis is essential and they should use good insect repellents, mosquito nets and protective covering. Limbs and body should be covered before dusk and early in the morning.

Counselling

This will depend the planned adventure activity. It should cover:

- ► vaccination
- ► dehydration
- ► avoidance of contaminated food
- ► drinking uncontaminated water
- ► infections from swimming in infested waters
- ► risks associated with trauma
- ► hypothermia
- ► altitude sickness.

Psychological problems

On expeditions, groups of people work together in very close proximity for some time, often in difficult circumstances. Although gregarious travellers enjoy such close contacts, the loner or those unaware of the complexities of a group psychology may struggle to cope (McIntosh, 1990). There is also a danger that small expeditions may fragment into smaller groups of two or three, risking the stability of the main party. Individuals can find themselves suddenly isolated and excluded from group activies (Pollit, 1986). Sometimes expedition members may be treated as pariahs when adversity and individual behaviour has created conflict. This can be seen in commercially organised trans-African expeditions among members not previously known to each other. They often leave the team halfway through the holiday as they are no longer able to tolerate close association with other members of the party.

When an individual joins an expedition, he/she becomes part of a group psychology which can be protective and supportive. However, if peer group support is withdrawn, this group psychology can become divisive and exclusive. Psychological pressure can be exerted to persuade an individual to conform to behaviour perceived as appropriate to the group's needs (Davis, 1993). Away from home and alternative support, these pressures can undermine personality, confidence and ego and are very threatening. There is psychological risk for those who will not, or cannot, participate as they may be ostracised and excluded from social interaction (Lucas, 1987). The reticent, retiring, introverted or depressed may be in, but not belonging to the expedition. Individual members of successful expeditions must be part of a cohesive, functioning group (McIntosh, 1992). This entails acceptance of unspoken rules for belonging, keeping to schedules and objectives, which often change during the expedition. Personal desires may have to be sublimated to ensure the success of the group. Many high climbing expeditions to the highest mountains have foundered on the inability of climbers to put the objectives of the group before their own personal ambitions.

Expedition members may be unprepared for the social intimacy which is an integral part of expeditioning. People may have to live close together in squalor, climatic extremes and under physiological stress. Habits, which are a minor annoyance in normal social situations, can become a major source of animosity. The smoker irritates the non-smoker, toilet and hygiene habits offend and personality conflicts can erupt if tents or refuges have to be shared for prolonged periods. Expeditions can bring out the best in the individual and the group, but they also have the potential to create conflicts which can be extremely damaging.

Doctors and nurses in travel clinics need to be aware of these psychological stresses and offer appropriate advice to help discourage such conflict (Calder and Wilder, 1989). If the possibility of conflict is likely to arise, this should be discussed with the client. Those who are suffering from depression or prefer their own company may be better advised to change their plans. Expedition doctors should be aware of potential problems and try to defuse the development of psychological conflicts. If an individual has overt personality problems, these may be recognised at the pre-expedition medical. Such individuals should then be excluded from the expedition (McIntosh, 1993a).

Potential problems can also be identified at pre-expedition 'shake-down' meetings and field outings arranged to test team members abilities. However, these trips have limitations unless the likely adverse expedition conditions can be re-created. As they are usually of short duration, it is not easy to find out how team members will react when confined together for longer periods. Raising awareness of potential group stressors in group members may help avoid later development of the psyche-destructive features of an expedition.

Most adventurers, back packers and trekkers accomplish their aims without suffering undue stress. If good advice, proper precautions and suitable vaccinations are taken, risks can be reduced significantly.

References

Barber S (1978) Drugs and doctoring for trans-Sahara travellers. *Br Med J* **295**: 404–6

Business Monitor and Use of Statistics (1992) *Overseas Travel and Tourism* (NQ6), Table 88. HMSO, London

Calder R, Wilder H (1989) Counselling the international traveller. *J Florida Med Ass* **76**: 379–85

Chatterjee S (1993) Differences in health behaviour of international travellers to Calcutta. *Proceeding of the Third International Conference of Travel Medicine*, Paris

Davis K (1969) *Group Performance*. Addison Wesley Publishing, Massachusetts: 25–8

Department of Health (1990) *Statements of Fees and Allowances* (The Red Book, London). HMSO, London

Forrester M (1987) *Survival*. McDonald, London

Gorman D (1992) Travel agents and the advice given to holiday makers. *Trav Med Int* **10**: 111–15

Green M, Kerr A, McIntosh I (1981) Acetazoleamide in acute mountain sickness: a double blind study. *Br Med J* **283**: 811–3

Hardy L (1998) Bilharzia: fighting the fluke. *Trav Med Int* **16**: 5–7

Illingworth R (1984) *Expedition Medicine and Planning Guide*. Scientific Publications, Oxford

Jauhar P, Weller M (1982) Psychiatric morbidity and time zone changes. *Br J Psychiatry* **140**: 321–35

Leech J (1978) The medicine of ocean yacht racing. *Br Med J* **2**: 1771–3

Lewis M (1965) Prevision and prevention. In: Edholm O, ed. *Exploration Medicine*. Wright, Bristol

Lucas GE (1987) Psychological aspects of travel. *Trav Med Int* **5**: 99–104

McIntosh IB (1990) The stress of modern travel. *Trav Med Int* **3**: 118–21

McIntosh IB (1991) Health hazards in water sports abroad. *Trav Med Int* **9**: 126–30

McIntosh IB (1992) Trials and tribulations of an expedition doctor. *Trav Med Int* **2**: 72–7

McIntosh IB (1993a) *Health Hazards in the High Risk Traveller*. Quay Publishing, Lancaster

McIntosh IB (1993b) Man on the mountains — the medical aspects. *Trav Med Int* **11**: 20–4

McIntosh IB, Prescott R (1986) Acetazolamide in presentations of AMS. *J Int Med Resources* **14**: 285–7

Mott A, Kinnersley P (1990) Overprescription of vaccine to travellers. *Br Med J* **300**: 25–6

Okhuysen P, Ericcson C (1992) Travellers diarrhoea prevention and treatment. *J Trav Med* **76**: 1357–72

Pollitt J (1986) The mind in travel. *Trav Med Int* **4**: 72–74

Reid D, Cossar JH (1994) Epidemiology of travel. *Br Med Bull* **49**(2): 265

Salisbury D, Begg T, eds. (1994) *Immunisation Against Infectious Diseases* (The Green Book). HMSO, London

Townend M (1998) The health of trekkers. *Trav Med Int* **16**: 8–11

Walker E (1994) *The ABC of Healthy Travel*, 4th edn. British Medical Association, London

8

Travel trauma and infection

International travel is a significant risk factor for accidents and the number of accidents sustained abroad by British travellers has doubled in recent years. Certain groups of travellers are more likely to suffer from trauma. These include; sportsmen and women, those between 20 and 29 years of age, travellers visiting developing countries for the first time, adventurers, backpackers and expeditioners. Trauma overseas in countries where emergency and medical care are rudimentary carries a high risk. Medical supplies and blood products may not be guaranteed as sterile or free from contamination. The injured are at risk from HIV and hepatitis infections.

By offering pre-travel consultations, practice nurses and doctors can assess a traveller's risk. Identifying the destination, the type of holiday and the activity planned, enables sufficient information to be gathered so that counselling can be tailored to the individual traveller. If the client has a history of sexually transmitted disease (STD), this may highlight a disregard for safe sexual practises when abroad. The risk of accident or unprotected sexual activity can be quantified and advice about appropriate hepatitis vaccination or use of condoms can be offered.

There is also a high risk from development of trauma-related infection. About a third of travel-related illness is due to trauma compared to 1.7% caused by infectious disease (Steffen, 1991). Those choosing vaccination with a bivalent hepatitis vaccine are protected if they sustain injury or contract liver infection.

Hepatitis B (HBV)

This infection occurs world-wide, with an estimated one in 2500 travellers developing symptoms after returning home. The virus is spread by carriers, or from the infected, during the incubation period or illness. It is 100 times more infective than HIV, the virus which causes AIDS. The World Health Organization has called for all countries to introduce routine hepatitis B vaccination and about 100 have already done so. Hepatitis B is the ninth most common cause of death world wide.

Prevalence

This varies markedly across the world, 5% of the population are carriers in Central and Eastern Europe, 20% of the population are carriers in parts of Africa, Asia and the Pacific and 12% of the hepatitis B infections recorded are contracted abroad (Steffen, 1995). The incidence is highest in adults living in squalor, in urban and rural areas. HBV is the third most common vaccine-preventable infection in travellers, after malaria and hepatitis A. Transmission is by skin penetration parenterally and sexually. Infectivity is blood-related, usually caused by:

- ▶ accidental inoculation procedures using inadequately sterilised needles and syringes, often by intravenous drug misusers sharing equipment

- ▶ blood to blood contact between people

- ▶ blood transfusion

- ▶ tattooing and acupuncture with dirty needles

- ▶ unprotected sexual contact, homosexual and heterosexual.

The virus is very stable and can survive in dried blood for up to one week. About 2–10% of those infected as adults become chronic carriers of the hepatitis virus, with hepatitis B surface antigen (HBsAG) persisting for longer than 6 months; 20–25% of hepatitis B carriers worldwide develop progressive liver disease.

Endemicity

High:	(prevalence 70–95%) Tropical Africa, Amazon Basin, South East Asia, parts of China and the Pacific Basin
Intermediate:	(prevalence 20–55%) Southern and Eastern Europe, Russia, Middle East, North Africa, Japan, India and parts of Central and South America

Symptoms

Hepatis B is usually of insidious onset with vague abdominal pains, nausea and vomiting and anorexia. These symptoms are all too familiar to tourists and are usually caused by the onset of travellers diarrhoea.

Fever is mild or absent and there may be arthralgia, a rash and, ultimately, jaundice.

Course of infection

Two thirds of those infected, develop clinical symptoms, half develop jaundice and 10% of those with clinical hepatitis do not fully recover, becoming chronic carriers. Two thirds of infections are asymptomatic and may never be diagnosed. The incubation period is 40–160 days so the presentation in Britiain is usually in returned international travellers. Hepatitis B is the only sexually transmitted infection which may be prevented by vaccination.

Vaccination

There are two types of immunisation product available. One is a vaccine which produces an immune response. The other is a specific immunoglobulin (HBIG), which provides passive immunity and can give immediate but temporary protection after accidental inoculation or contamination with antigen-positive blood. Combined active/ passive immunisation is recommended in those accidentally inoculated, or who have had eyes, mouth or fresh skin wounds contaminated with blood from a known HBsAG positive person.

Active immunisation with hepatitis B vaccine should be considered for long-stay travellers to endemic areas and 'at risk' groups working in tropical and sub-tropical areas. Immunisation is recommended in those at increased risk. This includes travellers to areas of high prevalence, especially health workers and those planning lengthy stays.

Hepatitis B vaccine contains the surface antigen (HBsAG) of HBV and there is a seroconversion rate of 99% in healthy adults after the standard vaccination regimen. It is well-tolerated. A multivalent HVB/HVA vaccine is available which provides protection against both infections.

Travellers at special risk

Travellers on expeditions, backpackers, recreational sports travellers and those living in rural areas benefit from twin protection. All are at risk of sustaining physical trauma and medical aid may be practised in unhygienic environments. Re-usable syringes and poor sterilisation procedures carry the risk of contamination and patient infection (Shandera, 1993).

Other travellers

Travellers from industrialised countries are increasingly choosing exotic destinations and avoiding conventional tourist haunts.

Vacations in:	1990	1994
Africa	493,000	720,000
Caribbean	208,000	328,000
South America	76,000	106,000

These numbers have increased even more dramatically in recent years. The rapid expansion of sea cruising is taking many first time cruise ship passengers to the Caribbean and undeveloped parts of Latin America, where there is high risk of contracting infection. They hire cars, bicycles, boats, water skiis and pedalos where potential trauma is a real threat. They forget that if an accident happens, emergency care could carry health risks from contaminated surgical equipment and blood products. They have a much higher risk of contracting hepatitis A and B infections. These infections are often acquired from medical and dental procedures in many countries visited by tourists and back-packers.

Unless their sexual behaviour places them in the high risk category, short-term tourist and business travellers are not normally at higher risk of infection. Back packers, adventurers and sportsmen or women may be in environments where the risk is greater, and should be vaccinated before going travelling. Hepatitis B vaccination is usually well-tolerated.

World travellers are frequently involved in road traffic accidents and may be admitted to hospital or clinics where sterilisation procedures are suspect. There is a high risk of HBV transmission in the developing countries of Asia and Africa. Homosexual and drug-abusing travellers are exposed to the risk of infection. Tourists who undergo tattooing, chiropody, dentistry or intrusive medical treatment are at risk, if instruments are inadequately sterilised. Mechanical transmission by biting insects, such as bed-bugs and mosquitoes may also spread the disease.

Studies of young tourists, who comprise the majority of the backpacker, sport, recreational and expeditioner groups, show that they are more likely to indulge in sexual activity on holiday and less likely to take precautions against infection. A quarter engage in sexual intercourse with new partners and condoms are used in less than half of these liaisons. The level of condom use is lowest in those having sexual intercourse with more than one partner.

Precautions

- ▶ pre-travel vaccination before visits to high risk areas of the world

- ▶ travellers should avoid penetration of the skin by objects previously in contact with the blood of others

- ▶ razor and needle-sharing should be avoided

- ▶ acupuncture, chiropody and dental treatment should be left until the return home

- ▶ condom protection with casual sexual relationships.

The possibility of infection must be kept in the mind if over zealous border officials insist on pre-entry cholera vaccination where syringes and needles may be contaminated.

Human immunodeficiency virus (HIV)

HIV is a world-wide problem, but choice of destination is less important in its occurrence than the behavioural patterns of travellers on business, tour or holiday. The World Health Organization has estimated that ten million adults are infected across the world, with a million infected in the USA. Sexual and drug-using behaviour rather than geographical location usually determine the risk to the traveller. However, in poor and developing countries, rural areas and up-country where disposable medical equipment is not available, the re-use of needles and syringes can cause blood contamination.

Road traffic accidents are common occurrences abroad. Emergency admission to hospitals and clinics in some countries in Africa and Asia have the added risk of transfusion with blood or blood products which have been inadequately screened or treated. After injury there may be reluctance to accept and it may be unwise to receive, blood from sources not known to be safe (Bewes, 1993).

Contamination of donor blood with the HIV virus, especially when donors are paid, may be impossible to rule out. One alternative is to accept blood only from 'safe' members of the travel group. Even this emergency aid measure can present unexpected problems.

Case history

In the pre-travel preparations for a climbing expedition to a remote part of the world with limited medical facilities, the medical officer decided that there was a risk that emergency care of any trauma casualties might mean transfusion with suspect blood. All the team members agreed to provide blood in an emergency and all were blood grouped before departure. In the event only minor trauma was sustained, although there was a narrow escape from a major traumatic incident.

On return to the UK, it later came to light that one of the team members — a universal donor — was HIV positive. This was not revealed at a confidential interview with the doctor or on the medical questionnaire completed before members were included in the expedition. In an emergency, team members might have been less at risk from locally available blood supplies than from a 'walking donor' on the expedition.

Travellers engaging in casual sexual behaviour are at high risk if in contact with people who might be HIV infected. They should be encouraged to use safe sexual practices and condoms. There is evidence that people when abroad are more likely to indulge in risky sexual behaviour. It has been suggested that 'touristhood' (Hanefors, 1994) has an effect on travellers in that they expand the operational and moral limits which they usually set for themselves. Some travellers feel 'incognito' abroad which encourages a sense of freedom to indulge in behaviour which they would not consider at home. Family and friends' stricter views on morality are not there to act as a restraint on the development of dubious sexual relationships. Barriers to casual sexual encounters and their attendant health risks are lowered.

Alcohol intoxication and drug abuse play major roles in the practice of unsafe sexual activity. Women indulging in casual sex were found to be consuming twice as much alcohol as a control group (Hellborg *et al*, 1995). Combined alcohol and drug abuse is a good predictor of sexual behaviour and indicates those who are more likely to indulge in unprotected sexual activity while abroad.

Re-use of medical equipment is common in many foreign countries, which are often unable to afford disposable equipment. Non-disposable syringes, needles and blood transfusion sets may be contaminated. In an emergency situation it is vital for the injured traveller or carer to ensure that nurses have been trained in good sterilisation and infection control procedures and that they are being applied. In many countries outside Western Europe, Northern America, Japan, Australia and New Zealand, adequate screening of donated blood may be the exception rather than the rule.

The World Health Organization now believes that most capital cities have at least one source of screened blood for transfusion. This is not always available to the injured traveller situated many miles from the capital. The risks of blood transfusion with infected blood remain high in many parts of the world and should be brought to travellers' attention at pre-travel consultations.

Dental, chiropody and acupuncture treatment is better left until the return home. Expeditioners, backpackers and sports people should be advised to travel with a well-equipped first aid kit, complete with disposable syringes and needles.

AIDS is on the increase and counselling about travel-related HIV infection should always be included in travel health clinic consultations. For the majority of travellers to countries of high or intermediate HAV endemicity, there is a much greater risk of contracting hepatitis A (HAV) infection. Steffen has estimated that susceptible travellers have a risk of 3–6 hepatitis A infections per 1000 months of travel in less developed countries. For 'off-beat' travellers this risk may be six times higher.

Little can be done for those suffering from HIV infection but vaccinations can now protect the majority of international tourists from travel-induced hepatitis. In terms of immunisable disease HepA and HepB infections are responsible for the greatest incidence of illness and death among travellers. HepA is the second most common disease contracted by unprotected travellers, after malaria. Expeditioners and backpackers often live in unhygienic conditions and they are at high risk of eating contaminated food and drinking infected water. Estimates suggest there is one case in every 50 for every month of stay depending upon the area visited.

Hepatitis A (HAV)

An inactivated hepatitis A vaccine is available with 100% protection one month after the first injection, with a booster ensuring longer protection. It offers protection for up to 10 years and will be welcomed by frequent travellers who have endured repeated gamma globulin injections. A blood test can check immunity to hepatitis A before giving the vaccine and its administration is particularly important for backpackers, frequent short-term travellers and those visiting rural areas in developing or third world countries.

Hepatitis A occurs endemically in many parts of the world especially where there is overcrowding, poor hygiene, inadequate water supplies and lack of sanitation. Travellers to areas outside industrialised Europe, North America, Australia and New Zealand can become infected and this unpleasant disease is often of prolonged duration.

Symptoms

The virus causes an acute inflammation of the liver and symptoms are fever, chill, fatigue, weakness, headache, aches and pains. This is followed later by nausea, vomiting anorexia, upper abdominal pain, jaundice, pigmented urine and light coloured stools.

In the young many infections are symptomless but jaundice can be severe and the illness prolonged. It may be followed by liver failure and coma. Although there is a low associated mortality, sufferers may be incapacitated for months. Mortality of 1.5% in people aged 64 years has been recorded by the UK Public Health Laboratory Service for those with fulminated hepatitis A infection. Data from the United States Department of Health and Human Services (1987) indicates that mortality rate may be up to 2.7% in those over 40 years of age. Underlying liver disease may have been a factor in some of these cases.

The viral incubation period is 35 weeks, with faecal shedding and infectivity greatest during this time. As many as 10% of hepatitis A patients are estimated to relapse (Gocke, 1986).

Incidence

Thirty million travellers from industrialised countries visit endemic areas annually. Perhaps as many as 40 percent of cases of hepatitis A are associated with recent international travel. HAV is, therefore, a major source of morbidity in travellers to developing countries with an estimated incidence among unprotected travellers as high as 20 per 1000 for each month of stay in an endemic area. The exact incidence is difficult to determine due to the occurrence of a high proportion of asymptomatic cases (Hadler, 1990).

HAV is often contracted by those travelling from areas of low to high prevalence, with all age groups susceptible. The risk of contracting the disease varies with the destination.

Endemicity

Very high:	Africa, parts of South America, the Middle East and South East Asia
High:	Amazon Basin of Brazil, China and Latin America
Moderate:	South and Eastern Europe

Risk of contracting hepatitis A

1.0	the non-traveller
2.6	travellers to Southern Italy
5.9	visitors to Eastern Europe and the Mediterranean
25.2	travellers to Africa, Asia, Southern and Central America

The risk also correlates with the mode of travel, the highest risk being among backpackers and travellers staying in primitive conditions.

In non-industrialised and developing countries, HAV infection is usually acquired sub-clinically in childhood but with improving standards of hygiene, children escape infection until infected clinically in young adulthood. It is spread from person to person by faecal/oral transmission caused by faecal contamination of food and water. Food-borne outbreaks are becoming more common in developed countries. Raw vegetables, fertilised with human night soil, and raw or poorly cooked shellfish grown in polluted waters, are recognised as highly infective sources of HAV.

Prevention of infection

Avoid eating uncooked shellfish and raw vegetables, and drink only sterilised water and milk.

The injection of human normal immunoglobulin (HNIG) consists of antibodies derived from pooled human serum. In recent years it has been used to give short-term protection, but the injection is often painful and this passive immunisation only protects short-term. As antibody levels decline from the time of the injection, frequent travellers must have repeat injections. A further disadvantage is that immunoglobulin cannot be administered at the same time or close to other live vaccines, such as poliomyelitis.

Inactivated vaccines are well-tolerated and highly immuno-genic. One month after vaccination with an initial dose, 95.6% of those given an initial dose have seroconverted. Geometric mean anti-HAV titres are approximately ten times higher than those occurring after passive immunisation more than sufficient to protect against hepatitis A infection. After a second dose one month later, seroconversion rises to 99.9% and the anti-HAV titres rise by about two thirds comparing favourably with passive immunity from immunoglobulin injection. The latter is a plasma product which gives only short-term protection for about five months, and its protection may decline with falling levels of immunity in developed countries. Two doses of vaccine should provide immunity for up to ten years.

It is cost effective to vaccinate regular international travellers to areas with poor standards of food and water hygiene. The 'Green Book' recommends protection for travellers to areas of moderate or high HAV endemicity, particularly if food hygiene and sanitation is poor. Active immunisation with vaccine is preferred, particularly with frequent travellers or for travellers who stay for more than three months. Travellers to all countries outside Northern or Western Europe, Northern America, New Zealand and Australia should be protected against hepatitis A infection. Older European and American adults, aged over 50 years of age, should be screened for antibodies before giving a vaccination as they may be immune.

Visitors to Africa, Asia and South and Central America, likely to be 'living rough', or travelling in areas of primitive sanitation and contaminated water supplies should always be considered for vaccination (Steffen, 1991).

References

Bewes P C (1993) Traumas and accidents. In: Behrens R, McAdam K ed. *Travellers Medicine*. The British Medical Bulletin, Churchill Livingstone, New York

Gocke DJ (1986) Hepatitis A revisited (editorial). *Ann Int Med* **105:** 960

Hadler S (1990) Global impact of hepatitis A virus infection changing patterns. *Proceedings of the International Symposium on Viral Hepatitis and Liver Disease*. Houston, Texas

Hanefors M (1994) Touristhood in the periphery of culture. In: Mardh P, ed. *Travel Medicine*. Scandinavian Association for Travel Medicine and Health. Upsala: 57–60

Hellborg D, Borendal M, Sikstrom B (1995) Comparison of women with cervical human papilloma virus.*Genitourinary Med* **71**: 88–91

Shandera W (1993) Travel and trauma. *J Wilderness Med* **4**: 40–61

Steffen R (1991) The epidemiologic basis for the practice of travel medicine. *Int Soc Trav Med* **2**: 10–15

Steffen R (1995) The epidemiological basis for the practice of travel medicine. *Second International Conferance of the International Society of Travel Medicine*. Atlanta, USA

US Department of Health and Human Services (1987) *Hepatitis Surveillance* (CDC), 51 18

9

Travel-related psychological trauma

Travel anxieties and stressors

Travel by road, rail and air for business or pleasure is an integral part of today's society. The risks of different methods of transport are quantifiable, and physical hazards can be identified and countered. Psychological trauma associated with travel is poorly appreciated and researched. Stress is common in national and international travel and routine stress tests on people who have recently been on holiday often reveal a significant negative effect. Long flights, congested roads, airports, seaports and railway stations increase stress levels. This chapter identifies some of these travel-related stressors, their impact on travellers and the role of the health professional in dealing with them.

International travel is frequent for many British citizens and 50 percent of the author's medical practice population admitted to travelling abroad annually. The majority of people travel on vacation, visiting countries throughout the world. Over 20 million journeys are made overseas each year by United Kingdom residents and in the last 40 years, the number travelling beyond Europe has multiplied 48 fold (Cossar *et al*, 1990).

Translocation — a known stressor

Travellers to destinations abroad may be exposed to health hazards, physical illness, trauma and disease. Many are affected by anxieties associated with translocation. This may vary from mild worry to more profound anxiety or severe fear. Profound anxiety and severe fears are well-researched but mild anxiety receives less attention. Such anxieties can spoil a holiday and can result in the development of fears or phobias which may inhibit further international travel.

Relocation is a recognised stressor (Lucas, 1987) and the psychological effects of a recent holiday can often be demonstrated on routine stress-testing. Britons leave the country by air and sea, by plane, ship and Eurostar. Each method has associated risks. Travellers are exposed to cultural differences, climate extremes and language barriers. They become anonymous, and are treated as inanimate objects to be moved from A to B by travel and transport operators.

Stressors

▶ transport difficulties, eg. delay

▶ congestion

▶ transmeridian disturbance

▶ time constraints

▶ uncertainty

▶ loss of personal control

▶ mass transit

▶ poor communications

▶ information overload.

These stresses occur when people are psychologically vulnerable (Pollit, 1986). Emotional upset is common and can be caused by the following (Black, 1993):

▶ cultural shock

▶ insecurity

▶ frustration

▶ psychological overload.

Travel-related anxieties and fears are common and Locke and Feinsad (1982) suggest that enjoyment of travel depends upon a predisposition to cope well with a variety of physical and psychological stresses. Their complexity has been recognised (Nahrwold, 1990; Fine, 1987) and they have been categorised as pre-travel and post-travel affective disturbances occurring during an absence from the home environment (Iljon and Iljoh, 1994). The anxiety caused by relocation suggests a third category, 'en route' psychological trauma. Arrival at the destination may also cause location anxieties.

Pre-travel anxieties

Pre-travel anxieties affect 'would-be' travellers and can cause travel phobias severe enough to prevent travel. Deep-rooted fears about flying, crossing under or over the water or travelling through long tunnels are common. In an island such as the United Kingdom, these fears can prevent travel outside the country. Travel stressors may mar the holiday, causing profound fear of the outward and return journeys and making travel a miserable experience.

Potential stressors can be induced by the method of travel, security procedures, customs checks, health hazards, language and cultural change (McIntosh, 1995). Anxiety ranges from mild agitation to morbid fear (Swanson *et al*, 1998).

Air travel-related anxiety

There is evidence that the degree of anxiety felt by the individual traveller does not equate with the actual risks of air travel (Moynihan, 1978). This also applies to anxieties about exposure to tropical illness and travel-related disease (McIntosh, 1996).

The prevalence of travel-related psychological disturbance has been poorly investigated but fear of flying is known to be common in travellers and non-travellers (Moynihan, 1978; Black, 1993). Harding and Mills, 1993) has identified anxieties related to flying as a passenger as:

▶ fear of heights

▶ fear of enclosed spaces

▶ being off the ground

▶ powerlessness

▶ proximity to others

▶ poor toilet access.

As the majority of the UK population leave the island by air, many are subject to these flying-related stressors (Steptoe, 1988).

How common are travel anxieties?

Estimates vary but population studies suggest that 10–13% of people have intense fears of flying (Agras, 1969; Burns and Thorpe, 1979; McIntosh, 1980a), 25% of Americans admit to fear of flying (Aronson, 1971), 30% of the Dutch admit to some measure of aerophobia (Van Gerwen, 1994) and 24% of Britons express anxieties about flying (McIntosh *et al*, 1996).

Doctors are frequently approached by those too afraid to travel and by potential travellers seeking medication to dispel anxieties relating to a forthcoming trip. Avoidance of travel can lead to business and family strife, stress and ill-health. McIntosh has studied the incidence of travel-related phobias in his medical practice population of surgery attenders. Fears of air travel, enclosed spaces, height and crowds were commonly reported and women were more likely to be subject to, or admit such fears (McIntosh, 1996).

The effects of translocation

Global travel alters routine and can effect the mental state of individual travellers. Congested motorways and airports, unpredictable and lengthy delays, communication problems, noise and fatigue can seriously disturb even the seasoned traveller. Stress tolerance levels are breached when disturbances, such as fog, accident or delay closes airport facilities. Relocation can confuse and disorientate the elderly and those unused to travel (McIntosh, 1990; 1992).

Travel survey

In a retrospective study, based on a 20% age and sex stratified quota sample of 1771 patients, aged 15 years and over, the anxiety-provoking features of international travel were investigated (McIntosh *et al*, 1996). The degree of anxiety experienced in travellers and those who had not travelled abroad was determined. Common travel worries identified were:

- ▶ flying
- ▶ illness while abroad
- ▶ travel sickness
- ▶ the climate
- ▶ infected food
- ▶ infected water
- ▶ pre-travel injections.

Worries about infected food and water predominate, with a third of travellers recording concern. One in four people express concern about flying, but men reported fewer anxieties than women. More non-travellers than travellers mentioned travel-related anxieties. Intensity of fear is greater for non-travellers in most travel anxieties. Travellers concerns about infected food, water and illness are usually justified by past experience.

Women report a greater prevalence of phobias and a greater intensity of fear than men. Allowing for the 'macho male' image which may prevent accurate recording of anxiety and phobia in men, there still appears a clear dominance in reported travel stressors among women. Women are particularly likely to admit to fear of flying, a fear disproportionate to the actual risk involved.

Anxieties about travel-related illness are largely unrealistic in terms of serious illness. Accidental trauma, especially in younger age groups, is the main cause of excess morbidity and death, but was a rarely reported anxiety. Although many health disturbances are reported by travellers most are relatively minor and in the majority of cases relate to traveller's diarrhoea. Fear expressed about takeoff and landing are more realistic as this is the time when air accidents are most likely to occur. Anxieties concerning baggage retrieval are also justified and may result from experience. Luggage in transit by air often does go astray. Flight delays are particularly stressful (Straddling, 1994) and technical problems with aircraft can trigger phobia.

Pre-flight distress

Pre-flight and in-transit stress may increase the risk of cardiac problems in air travellers. Cardiac incidents account for 15% of in-flight emergencies and more than half of in-flight deaths (Roscoe, 1996). However, airport physicians suggest that the wait in the airport may be more hazardous to the health of travellers than the flight, with arrivals more at risk than departures. (Neumann, 1996). The Federal Aviation Administration in America has recently noted that there are now 15 medical emergencies per day on US airlines compared with three per day in 1986. It is believed that some of these may be associated with stress created by handling baggage, flight delays, customs inspections and security clearances.

Fear-induced hyperventilation is the most frequently encountered cause of distress during commercial air travel. Episodes of over-breathing are recognised by airline staff who offer support and counselling. They are often triggered by an accumulation of events before and during the flight. Pre-flight congestion in the departure hall will test the agoraphobic beyond endurance; closure of aircraft doors causes panic in the claustrophobic; dining, in the close confines of an aircraft cabin facing strangers, disturbs the social phobic and flying unsupported in space is a trial for those with aircraft phobia. These phobics can quickly panic and hyperventilate (a sign of psychological distress).

Case history

The doors on the aircraft were closed, departure was announced and after some delay the captain regretfully announced that there was a fault in the computer which they were trying to rectify. One hour later passengers were told that the fault could not be traced but that they could fly using the other two computers on board. There was another delay of an hour and then a further message that the second computer was misbehaving but it would be put right. Ultimately this computer had to be replaced and 2 hours later the flight was ready to depart. Passengers had been kept locked in a very warm aircraft, fastened in their seats and, at this stage, a teenage girl became hysterical, hyperventilated and collapsed. On recovery she refused to fly. Despite the efforts of the crew she and her family were disembarked, causing further delay to the departure of the aircraft.

On another occasion, a long haul aeroplane set off for India. After half an hour an engine fault forced a return to the departure airport. Three hours later it took off again. Not long into the flight a fire occurred in one engine, which was promptly extinguished. Emergency escape procedures were rehearsed and the incident resulted in a further return to the airport. Passengers were disembarked and taken to another airfield and another aeroplane Several refused to fly on. One became severely aircraft phobic and could not fly again. As a business-man this was catastrophic for his career and, ultimately, he lost his job.

Thirty years ago the passenger could stroll up to the airline counter 15 minutes before the flight, buy a ticket and he/she and his/her luggage would be weighed. There was a few yards walk out to the aerodrome and the aircraft, and boarding and takeoff followed within minutes. Aeroplanes were parked close to entry and departure lounges, concerns about security were minimal and the general mood was one of relaxed informality. Now huge airports, a multiplicity of gates, interminable walkways, impersonal employees and tight security all intimidate the traveller. Aggravation, congestion, information overload and noise assault waiting clients. Passengers, some who fail to cope, are forced to overcome an endless succession of barriers before reaching the aircraft.

Relocation — psychological problems

Long haul transmeridian flights cause desynchronisation of circadian rhythm with readjustment taking some days after arrival at the destination. A study of people admitted from Heathrow airport to a nearby psychiatric unit, found a significant increase in depression on flights from east to west whereas the incidence of hypomania increased by a similar ratio when going in the opposite direction. Rapid time zone change appears to precipitate affective illness in those predisposed (Jauhar, 1982). This may be related to the phase retardation in the sleep/wake cycle which occurs in east to west transmeridian travel.

Depressed patients cannot cope with rapid transit and environmental change and their condition is likely to deteriorate further if they travel globally. Such patients should be discouraged from international travel and, in particular, from sea cruising. Cruise ships can be lonely places for the non-gregarious and the depressed. Excess alcohol may be used as a prop and, rather than offer a solution to their problems, it can increase the risk of suicide.

Keeping on the move and travelling are early signs of mania. Euphoria and elation are poor travelling companions and those with hypomania are a major problem on aircraft or in small groups. Their behaviour stands out on cruise ships and, even if amusing, can put other passengers at risk during small craft transfer. Brain cell damage in early Alzheimer's disease causes personality change and minor memory loss. Although not obvious in the home environment, it becomes rapidly apparent during foreign travel. Passengers with their senses intact and a good memory can become disorientated in large airports, those with organic brain disease become totally confused. Elderly people with early senile dementia lose all sense of direction in airports and stations and often find they have forgotten the name of their cruise ship and where it is berthed. In a foreign port where the language and people are unknown, this can be a devastating experience.

Case history

> *An elderly person with Parkinson's disease and mild memory loss caused by encroaching dementia was determined to visit his family in Australia. He travelled alone and had a successful holiday. During the return there were flight delays and re-routing. He arrived at Heathrow airport early in the morning suffering from jet lag and fatigue. Completely disorientated he wandered round the airport so confused that he missed his connection. At midnight his disorientation and confusion were recognised by a patrolling policemen and he was taken to the medical centre. The staff organised his overnight stay and onward flight the next day. The following morning his confusion had gone but at home a worried family, waiting his arrival the previous day, feared for his safety. Very relieved at his final homecoming, they vowed to discourage further long distance travel.*

Safe arrival at the destination is not always the relaxing experience shown in tourist brochures. The culture shock of visits to Asia, Africa and South America can be intensely distressing and may discourage further travel abroad. Abject poverty, the gulf between the 'haves and have nots' and the differences in social structures in developed and developing countries are too disturbing and challenging for some.

Poverty, racism, religious extremism and hostility to tourists can horrify the traveller. They may react by withdrawing from contact with the local population, isolating and insulating themselves in the safety of tourist groups and hotels. Fear of black or coloured people or of indigenous populations prevents many first-time travellers from leaving the tour coach. They visit only well-known sights or night clubs. Fears of physical aggression and personal injury are common, especially in women travellers. Theft and assault on tourist beaches and holiday resorts does occur, but these fears are often exploited by state and tour agencies to maximise profits within the holiday complex. Anxious tourists concerned for their safety are herded to in-house entertainment and inclusive tours where there is little contact with the local population. With a few exceptions, risk of physical harm to a tourist abroad is low and related anxieties, although protective, are unrealistic.

Travel group stresses

Protected by the travel agency, the tour guide and cocooned in the travel programme, people are treated like packages. They are wrapped in group psychology and accept group rules. They follow pre-selected schedules, join in events and accept changes unquestioningly. They become part of a gregarious whole. However, for those who will not or cannot accept such a group mentality, there are psychological dangers. They may become isolated and excluded from the social interaction, and ostracised by other group members. Clients who are reticent, retiring, introverted or depressed may feel that they do not belong, and the security, which they expected to find within the group they have joined, is lacking. Actively belonging to, or being separated from a group can make or mar a holiday.

On the fringe of a group or expedition, the individual may suffer the loneliness experienced by the solo traveller. Clients travel alone out of necessity for business reasons, as backpackers or tourists. For them congested departure points, such as airport concourses or railway stations can be intimidating. Solo travellers can suffer feelings of separation, such as home sickness, solitude and isolation and may use alcohol as a prop to keep such feelings at a distance.

A considerable number of travellers and non-travellers are afflicted by anxieties of sufficient intensity to provoke behavioural changes and avoidance, which are phobic in nature.

The role of the health professional

In-transit stressors have been poorly researched and are rarely considered by travel agents and travel health clinic personnel (Hill and Behrens, 1996). They may be the source of sufficient psychological stress to cause cardiological or stress-related ill health later in the journey. Travel agents rarely address these issues with clients (Gorman and Smyth, 1992). The travel health clinic has been shown to be effective in diminishing ill health in travellers (Reed *et al*, 1995). The travel industry's role in promoting good health in travellers has been recognised and collaboration between the industry and community travel medicine clinics has been recommended (Steffen and DuPont, 1994). A combined effort to minimise known health stressors might lead to healthier travel. Pre- and post-travel-related stress is poorly addressed and patients reporting travel anxieties and phobias may not receive appropriate advice from their general practitioner. It has been shown that doctors and travel health clinic personnel often fail to provide advice to intending travellers (Straddling, 1994; Keystone *et al*, 1994).

The role of travel health clinics should include advice and counselling on all aspects of the impact of travel on the individual (McIntosh, 1980b). The travel-related anxieties, felt by many people about food and water hygiene abroad, could be used to persuade travellers into taking sensible precautions to prevent traveller's diarrhoea. Travel health education should highlight the risks of contracting gastrointestinal infection in areas where standards of food hygiene are low or non-existent. Travellers can be advised to avoid high risk foods, such as shellfish. If choice is limited they should boil suspect food and make sure it is thoroughly cooked. Fruit should be peeled, by themselves, after carefully washing their hands, and water should be sterilised.

The effects of travel stressors should be considered. This is essential for those with existing clinical conditions, such as cardiac disease. These can be aggravated by undue stress during international travel. Unrealistic fears and phobias identified at pre-travel consultations should be dealt with. They can be allayed or diminished by proper counselling and may be cured by behavioural therapy and hypnotherapy prior to departure, if there is sufficient time. General practitioners with an interest in travel health and therapy may, themselves, treat patients or refer them on to a behavioural therapist or psycholgist.

Treatment of travel anxieties

Surgery consultations may reveal that a patient is unable to face the prospects of leaving the United Kingdom due to travel fears or phobias. Many of those who refuse to travel do so from fear and anxiety rather than lack of finance. Effective therapies are available. Behavioural therapy (France and Robson, 1986), cognitive therapy (Greco, 1989), hynotherapy (McIntosh, 1992) and neurolinguistic programming techniques (McDermott, 1997) can help patients to come to terms with their fears. No one should be denied access to global travel by psychological inhibitions through lack of treatment.

There will always be some anxiety associated with international travel, even if it is only concerned with reaching the airport on time. The increasing number of international travellers, bigger airports, larger aeroplanes and cruise ships, terrorism and hijack are all factors that increase the relocation stress which affects the global traveller.

All health professionals, particularly those working in travel, should be aware of the psychological impact of global translocation and transportation on the individual, and should be prepared to offer counselling, advice and therapy to mitigate its effects.

Travel clinic counselling

- ► consider the psychological stresses of potential travel at pre-travel counselling, particularly in the elderly and those with chronic disease

- ► suggest direct routes, upgrading of seats, use of executive lounges, pre-travel seat booking for those embarking on long haul flights

- ► identify travellers and non-travellers with travel-related phobias and organise behavioural, cognitive or hypno-therapy for its treatment

- ► consider the effect of travel and translocation on the depressed person who should be discouraged from solo travel and sea cruising

- ► discuss the effects of jet lag and how these can be minimised

- ► use traveller's realistic anxieties about contaminated food and water to reinforce education on food and hygiene precautions

- ► discourage the use of alcohol and tranquillisers to deal with travel fears and anxieties.

Aircraft fear, phobias and their management

Sixteen million, five hundred thousand people leave the UK by air annually (CSO, 1988). Whether on business or holiday, travellers must cope with transport problems and transmeridian disturbance during relocation (Lucas, 1897). For the psychologically vulnerable, this can cause considerable stress (Pollit, 1986). Travel worries, fears and phobias are common and can provoke emotional scenes. Before departure, travellers may be close to their maximum level of stress tolerance (McIntosh, 1990).

It has been suggested that safety and enjoyment of travel depends largely on adequate preparation and a predisposition to cope well with change, physical and psychological stresses (Locke and Feinsod, 1982). Air travel, or potential travel, can be psychologically traumatic and some clients will refuse to fly. For others anxiety is caused by pre-flight security checks of baggage and personal effects, which may remind travellers of the risks of hijack and in-flight explosion. Delayed flight departures and lack of information can make travellers feel unimportant and apprehensive, eroding self-confidence.

Flying is traumatic for many passengers and Greco (1989) has suggested that this is because it means confronting innate fears, such as fear of heights, falling, enclosed spaces and social crowding. Howards *et al* (1983) point out that fear of flying is not a unitary phenomenon and identifies four 'source fears' of crashing, heights, confinement and instability/turbulence. Awareness of these fears is essential when considering appropriate treatment.

People normally try to make sense of the visual and auditory input from their environment. Strange in-flight noises, such as engine, wing flap and air conditioning noises, confuse them and they lack the technical knowledge to identify the cause of these noises and exclude a potential threat. This results in increased tension and further insecurity. Calming and relaxation techniques can be remarkably effective in treatment of aeroplane related fears and phobias.

Travel fears vary from mild anxieties to severe phobias. Some cross the Diagnostic and Statistical Manual of Mental Disorders (DSM 4; 1994) diagnostic categories of anxiety disorder ranging from panic disorder to severe phobic state. They can present as simple and common 'In-flight Stress Malaise' (Chapman, 1995) or an overt phobia that prevents clients from travelling.

Phobia

Phobia causes anxiety and fear out of all proportion to what is regarded as rational. It is involuntary, cannot be explained or reasoned away and leads to avoidance behaviour. There are four elements to a phobia:

a cognitive element	*subjective fear*
behavioural response	*avoidance of the feared situation*
physiological manifestations	*tachycardia, palpitations, hyperventilation*
a social component	*disruption of normal living*

For those apprehensive about flying, anxieties are not resolved by safe arrival at the destination. They brave the outward flight but will continue to worry about the return journey. Although common, travel-related anxieties, stressors, fears and phobias have been poorly researched and their prevalence has not been properly established. The majority of travellers who suffer worries and phobias appear to be women, and 2.8% of these worries are travel phobias. Women are more prepared to admit to the problem than men and are more likely to seek treatment (Burns and Thorpe, 1979). In his general medical practice, McIntosh (1980) states that 16% of those over 16 years of age recorded the presence of a phobia with 13% of this sub-group reporting fear of flying. The female to male preponderance was 2:1. Other reports suggest that one in ten adults admit to intense fear of flying. Flying phobia was the second most common travel related phobia reported by patients (McIntosh *et al*, 1996). Of those, 29% who had not recently travelled abroad, admitted to major fears about air travel, a quarter had never travelled overseas and in many cases this was because their phobia prevented them from doing so. The avoidance response of phobic behaviour is often a bar to foreign travel. An increase in numbers of travellers who fly has led to a steady increase in those seeking treatment for phobia.

Fear of flying is disproportionate to the actual risk of a hazardous event occurring. Air travel is a relatively safe transport method. The intensity of anxieties experienced by non-travellers restricts their geographic mobility and impairs their quality of life. Over half the adult population travels abroad in a three year period and international travel is common for the majority of the British population. Irrational fear, which prevents such travel, can overshadow family relationships and limit employment opportunities if world travel is a necessary part of an employee's role.

Case history A

> *A woman presented at the end of a surgery session one evening, very distraught and demanding a medical certificate for an airline as she was unfit to travel. It transpired that she had sold her business and house and was emigrating to South Africa to marry. She had a longstanding fear of flying but, in the excitement of the wedding and removal preparations, her fear had been thrust aside. It had surfaced a few days ago. As time for her departure drew closer, so her apprehensions grew. She was now intent on avoiding exposure to the threat of air travel.*
>
> *There was little time to help her but after counselling she agreed to hypnotherapy which was very effective. She travelled by air later that week and has travelled successfully for many years since.*

Case history B

> *A business man came to the surgery in considerable agitation. His new managerial job involved much United Kingdom travel. Over recent months his fear of flying had become a phobia. He had been avoiding air travel and going to London by train and car. This was time consuming and exhausting and was ruining his work. He had been given an ultimatum — travel by air or resign!*
>
> *With the help of simple behavioural and hypnotherapy, he resolved his fears and moved up the promotion ladder to a senior management post.*

Phobic travellers often seek treatment but many of the travelling public suffer from apprehension and anxiety which has attracted little professional attention. Varying degrees of anxiety are expressed concerning travel-related events, which are peripheral to the actual flight. These may be significant stressors in the elderly, those suffering from chronic illness and for those with existing cardiovascular disability. The physical demands of air transit for the frail and elderly passenger are considerable. Carrying heavy luggage through arrival and departure lounges, prolonged standing, long walkways and steep stairways are common at most international airports.

In a self-report study of airport and aircraft-related anxieties and stessors, women were found to be more apprehensive about flying than men (Swanson *et al*, 1998). The severity of women's distress also appeared to be greater than in men and they developed more somatic problems related to air travel than men. They showed a strong association between overall anxiety experienced and the somatic symptoms usually asociated with stress, eg. tachycardia, tachypnoea and muscle tension.

The highest risk in flying is during take-off and landing and is a legitimate anxiety. However, flight delays and baggage reclaim, where there is no risk to safety, are also stressful. Flight delay caused anxiety in 50% of passengers and this stress was exacerbated by:

► lack of information

► time lost

► inconvenience

► loss of personal control

► communication difficulties.

For some travellers, this is also the time when they are particularly vulnerable to stress. They either anticipate travel stress or respond to it, as follows:

► 33% drink alcohol to relax

► 5% resort to prescribed or OTC medication

► 20% use relaxation and distraction techniques to combat anxiety

Health professionals should encourage travellers who drink or take drugs, to use behavioural conditioning and hypnotherapeutic techniques instead. Although taking alcohol or drugs reduces the symptoms, they do little to treat the underlying psychological problem and are poor coping mechanisms for dealing with travel-related stressors (McIntosh, 1990)

Airlines and travel agencies could initiate measures to reassure clients and diminish stressful situations when there are onward travel delays. Ensuring that additional information is provided, improving communication and better management prodedures could reduce the stress caused by delay and baggage retrieval. Health professionals should use behavioural therapy to treat clients with anxieties about flying, rather than prescribe medication. They should also be aware that air travel is a particular cause of physical stress for elderly people and additional psychological distress can precipitate in-transit morbidity. Stress management and counselling could be offered at the pre-travel health clinic assessment consultation.

The management role

Many severe travel anxieties and phobias will respond to therapy. A greater professional awareness of travel stressors, their intensity and the potential for cure benefits many patients. Appropriate therapy should be initiated either by a family practitioner or on referral. Intense fears of flying should be identified and treated. Most practitioners will at some time have had a distraught patient attend the surgery a day or two before a flight, stating that they cannot face an imminent journey. To the dismay of the family or friends, they try to cancel the holiday. Other clients may ask for tranquillisers to be prescribed in the run up to departure. During routine consultation, some will admit to being phobic to ships, aeroplanes or crowds. They cannot contemplate leaving home even though they would like to travel abroad. Many can be helped with appropriate therapy.

In travel clinics, much pre-travel counselling is done by the practice nurse. The pre-travel assessment protocol should include questions about travel anxieties and fears, which identify potential problems. The nurse can offer simple advice to minimise known travel stressors and can suggest simple relaxation techniques to reduce travel tension (McIntosh, 1990). Behavioural therapy, autogenic training, neurolinguistic programming and hypnotherapy can be used to treat phobic clients. Simple anxieties respond well to stress management techniques and most fears and phobias will respond to behavioural therapy (McIntosh, 1992).

Fear is normal and an essential part of everyday living. It is a response to a real or imagined threat, with a behavioural element which is often pronounced. Fears range from mild to intense and the latter is usually described as a phobia. This is a morbid response, disproportinate to the causative stimulus, which often causes sufferers to structure their lives in such a way as to avoid fear-provoking situations, ie. air travel.

Behavioural modification techniques

Based on exposure to a feared situation
1. Imaginational exposure in the presence of a therapist
2. *In vivo* exposure — with or without a therapist
3. Self-hypnosis
4. Self-statement training
5. Neuro-liguistic programming using imagery

In the weeks prior to travel, cognitive, behavioural therapy using desensitisation techniques is widely used by clinical psychologists to treat phobics. The principle is to keep exposing the patient to the situation which causes distress until they get used to it. Attempts are then made to to extinguish the fear by relating it to a pattern of behaviour which provokes no anxiety. Most respond well to this treatment but the process is time consuming.

A hierarchy of anxiety-provoking situations leading to the actual flight is created with the patient's co-operation. The patient imagines him/herself in the feared situation and experiences the responses usually evoked in that situation. He/she is 'talked through' the experience by the therapist who offers relaxation and calming suggestions. A typical hierarchy could involve the drive to the airport, passage from check-in to air-side, boarding the aircraft and takeoff. Imaginational exposure is used by most therapists. Some airlines offer therapy courses which terminate with a short flight to clearly demonstrate the patient's escape from the prevailing phobia.

Hypnotherapists have used similar methods, often with quicker curative responses. The use of hypnosis for phobias is well established and therapy seems to be helped by trance induction. Implosion or flooding techniques, the opposite of graduated desensitisation, either in or out of trance, can work successfully in a single session. Hypnotherapy and neurolinguistic programming techniques can work quickly and are useful for people who present shortly before planned departure dates.

Desensitisation

Involves: patient instruction

creation of a hierarchy of anxiety provoking events

graduated exposure to the feared event

concurrent contrasting experience, eg. relaxation

positive reinforcement

Flooding

Involves: patient instruction

non-graduated, uninterrupted exposure to aversive stimuli with avoidance prevention

no contrasting or distracting techniques

positive verbal reinforcement

This technique seems particularly effective when carried out with the patient in a hypnotherapeutic trance.

Neurolinguistic programming (NLP)

NLP, where the individual imagines scenarios related to the threatening situation, can be very effective in treating anxieties and phobias. The technique can also work very quickly and be practised in the conventional surgery consultation. NLP was developed by Richard Bandler, a computer scientist and John Grinder a linguistics lecturer who studied the work of Milton Ericson, Virginia Satir and Fritz Perls in hypnotherapy, family and gestalt therapy. They identified a common communication link which all three used with their patients and this appeared to be the most effective part of their therapy.

The system they developed is based on how people actually think and the usefulness to them of what they actually think about. It is a person-centred approach to care. NLP practitioners' 'fast phobic' cures depend upon dissociation and then reversal of the associated memory of the feared incident in the imagination. They use 'anchoring' where a resourceful state is associated with a specific touch and the resourceful feelings are then taken into imagined future situations likely to be anxiety provoking. The patient then uses these new resources to extinguish apprehension and fear. Doctors who practice these behavioural techniques are impressed by the speed and permanence of change in patient response.

GPs have often prescribed anxiolytics for air travel phobic people. Prescription of a tranquilliser may be tempting for a harassed family doctor. Some precribe beta blockers which help to control peripheral sympathetic responses such as palpitations. However, drugs do nothing to cure the phobia and are better avoided.

The phobic person who wants to travel can be treated. Doctors who are interested and appropriately skilled are able to treat their clients during consultations or at the travel health clinic. Others should refer the patient promptly for the services of psychologists, behavioural therapists and hypnotherapists. Drug medication should be avoided as this only treats the symptom and not the underlying disorder.

Stressors and phobias can ruin holidays and sabotage employment opportunities. They should be identified pre- and post-travel in clinics and routine consultations. Most patients will gratefully accept offers of treatment. Therapy will free them from stress and fear, allowing them to embark successfully upon world travel.

Incidence of phobias in the population

Not definitely known	
Community surveys suggest	5–10% in over 65 year olds 3% of general population 1 year prevalence of social phobia: 5% life-time risk: 13%
UK studies	1 in 10 adults has been reported as having a flying phobia (Steptoe 1988) 3% of all phobias reported by women are travel phobias (Burns and Thorpe, 1979)
In a 20% sample of a general practice population:	27% admitted to fears and phobias 17% would have accepted treatment (McIntosh *et al*, 1996)

1.	Air travel or the thought of an air journey can be psychologically terrifying for some people. Phobias deter others from travelling abroad and spoil holidays and business trips. Aircraft phobia is a travel-related fear for which potential travellers seek treatment. It prompts behavioural responses and avoidance disproportionate to risk to life and limb
2.	Aircraft-related phobias are simple to treat using behavioural modification techniques. Phobics can be freed from fear and successfully travel the world

Key points

1.	Travel phobia — a degree of anxiety and fear out of all proportion to the evoking stimulus
2.	There are physiological, behavioural cognitive and social components to phobias
3.	Flying phobia is the second most common travel-related phobia reported
4.	As many as 1 in 10 adults may have an intense fear of flying
5.	Travel phobias respond well to treatment
6.	Behavioural modification techniques are commonly used to treat phobias
7.	Hypnotherapy can be very effective in phobia treatment
8.	Neurolinguistic programming techniques appear to work quickly in the treatment of travel phobias

References

Agras S, Sylvester D, Oliveau D (1969) The epidemiology of common fears and phobias. *Comprehen Psychiatry* **10**: 151–67

American Psychiatric Association (1994) *Diagnostic and Statistical Manual of Mental Disorders*. DSM 4th edn. AMA, Washington DC

Aronson ML (1971) *How to Overcome Your Fear of Flying*. Hawthorne, New York

Black J (1993) Travellers ploys — how to stay in one piece. *Trav Med Int* **11**(1): 8–13

Burns L, Thorpe G (1979) Fears and phobias. *J Int Med Res* **5**(Suppl 1): 132–9

Chapman P (1995) In-flight emergencies. *Trav Med Int* **13**: 171–3

Chief Scientist's Office (1988) *Travel Trends*. HMSO, London: 18

Cossar JH, Reid D, Fallon RJ *et al* (1990) A cumulative review of studies on travellers, their experience of illness and the implications of these findings. *J Infection* **21**: 27–42

Fine R (1987) Geography and the super-ego. A contribution to psycho-geography and the psychology of travel. *J Psycho-History* **1**: **14**(4): 351–62

France R, Robson M (1986) *Behaviour Therapy in Primary Care — A Practical Guide*. Croom Helme, London

Gorman D, Smyth B (1992) Travel agents and advice giver to travellers. *Trav Med Int* **9**: 111–15

Greco TS (1989) A cognitive-behavioural approach to fear of flying. A practitioners guide. *Phobia Pract Res J* **2**(1): 3–15

Harding RM, Mills JF (1993) *Aviation Medicine*, 3rd edn. BMJ Publishing Group, London

Hill DR, Behrens RH (1996) A survey of travel clinics throughout the world. *J Trav Med* **3**: 46–51

Howards W, Murphy S, Clarke J (1983) Nature and treatment of fear of flying. *Behav Ther* **14**: 557–67

Iljon Foreman E, Iljon Z (1992) Highwaymen to hijackers — a survey of travel fears. *Trav Med Int* **12**(4): 145–51

Jauhar P, Weller M (1982) Psychiatric morbidity and time zone changes. *Br J Psychiatry* **140**: 321–35

Keystone J, Dismukas R, Sawyer L, Kozarsky E (1994) Inadequacies in health recommendations for international travellers. *J Trav Med* **1**: 72–8

Locke S, Feinsod F (1989) Psychological preparation for young travellers. *Adolesc* **17**(68): 815–9

Lucas G (1987) Psychological aspects of travel. *Trav Med Int* **3**: 99–104

McDermott P (1997) Fears, phobias and neurolinguistic programming. *J Br Soc Med Dent Hypnosis* **17**: 47–9

McIntosh IB (1980a) The incidence, management and treatment of phobias in a group medical practice. *Pharmaceut Med* **1**(2): 77–82

McIntosh IB (1980b) Setting up a GP travel health clinic. *Trav Med Int* **13**(4): 148–51

McIntosh IB (1989) Travel considerations in the elderly. *Trav Med Int* **7**: 69–72

McIntosh IB (1990) Stress and coping in travel. *Trav Med Int* **8**(3): 118–21

McIntosh IB (1992a) Treating travel phobias with hypnotherapy. *J Br Soc Med Dent Hypnosis* **1**: 28–30

McIntosh IB (1992b) *Travel and Health in the Elderly*. Quay Publishing, Lancaster

McIntosh IB (1995) Travel phobias. *J Trav Med* **2**: 99–100

McIntosh IB, Power K, Reed J (1996) Prevalence intensity and sexual differences in travel-related stressors. *J Trav Med* **3**: 96–102

Moynihan B (1978) *Airport International*. Pan Books, London: 14

Nahrwold MI (1990) Fear of flying, or, an anaesthetised patient is not an aeroplane. *Anaesthesiol Rev* **14**(5): 68–72

Neumann K (1996) Turbulence in the air — flight-related health problems. *Trav Med Int* **14**: 3

Pollit J (1986) The mind and travel. *Trav Med Int* **4**: 72–4

Reed J, McIntosh IB, Power K (1995) Travel illness and the family practitioner. *J Trav Med* **1**: 192–7

Roscoe AH (1996) Medical fitness for air travel. *Trav Med Int* **14**: 200–6

Steffen R, DuPOnt H (1994) Travel mediccione. Whats that? *J Trav Med* **1**: 1–3

Steptoe A (1988) Managing flying phobia, editorial. *Br Med J* **296**: 25

Straddling H (1994) A travel clinic audit. *Trav Med Int* **12**(3): 83–8

Swanson V, McIntosh IB, Power K (1998) Air travel anxieties in health professionals. *Scott Med J* (In press)

Van Gerwen L (1994) *Holland Herald – KLM in Flight Publication*: 51

10

Travel-related physiological trauma

World travellers are exposed to health risks from physical, psychological and physiological trauma. Physiological trauma includes disturbance to circadian rhythm as a result of crossing time zones, exposure to low partial pressure of oxygen in aeroplanes and high altitude environments and over-stimulation of the labyrinth sensory organ in travel motion. This can cause jet-lag, hypoxia, acute mountain sickness (AMS) and travel sickness.

Travel sickness

Motion sickness includes: sea and air sickness, car and air sickness and can extend to symptoms of nausea and sickness affecting those who ride camels and elephants, or explore space. It is a debilitating but usually short-lived disorder. When man is exposed to atypical forces in the environment, the harmony of the balance system sensory input can be disrupted. The degree of motion sickness experienced can range from mild discomfort to severe sickness. Only deaf mutes with non-functioning labyrinths are known to be immune.

The disorder was well-known to ancient Greek mariners who called the condition nauxia — the precursor of the English word, nausea. Julius Caesar is recorded as having suffered grievously from the illness when crossing to England from France. Lord Nelson had to fight off sea-sickness on each departure from port. Lawrence of Arabia experienced motion sickness on his long camel rides and many soldiers of the British invasion force on D-day suffered sea sickness as they crossed the English Channel. Early astronauts experienced motion sickness on their space voyages.

Prevalence of motion sickness

In the normal population :

> 5% will suffer severely
>
> 5% will be hardly affected
>
> 90% will suffer moderately
>
> 70% of ship passengers may be affected in rough weather (Velimirovic, 1990)
>
> 5% of those afflicted will not adapt to sea travel unless the high seas abate

A consistent research finding is that women are more susceptible to the illness than men. They have a higher susceptibility near the onset of menstruation, or during pregnancy. Susceptibility is an enduring trait and, although there is some reduction in susceptibility with age, many older sea going passengers will succumb in stormy weather and high seas.

Effects of age

- ▶ incidence of travel sickness decreases between the ages of 21 and forty
- ▶ incidence increases to a maximum between 12 and 21 years
- ▶ travel sickness is rare before the age of 2 years, although very young babies can be affected
- ▶ age does not confer immunity to disruptions of normal motion.

Sopite syndrome

The mildest form of motion sickness is known as the Sopite syndrome, and symptoms are limited to:

- ▶ some gasping
- ▶ drowsiness
- ▶ decreased interest in the local environment
- ▶ a tendency towards physical inactivity.

At the other extreme there are reports of sickness occurring as soon as passengers mount the gangway of the ship.

Cause

Motion sickness is a physiological vertigo which might be more appropriately referred to as motion maladaption syndrome. The exact cause is still not understood despite much research, particularly that related to the space programme. The symptoms are the penalty paid by those who go beyond the specifications for which humanity is designed in the evolutionary process (Oosterveld, 1997). Many hypotheses have been suggested with respect to the origin of motion sickness but none offer a full explanation. The illness appears to arise from intense stimulation of the labyrinthine sense organs over a period of time, in a manner to which the body is not accustomed. Irritation of labyrinthine receptors by vertical and oscillatory movements transmits impulses directly or by way of the vestibular nuclei, through the cerebellum to the centre of the vomiting reflex (Guyton, 1976). Motion-related nausea sometimes occurs without vomiting. This may be the result of a lesser labyrinth stimulation than that which causes impulses to reach the vomit centre.

The incoming sensory irritation also involves the vagus, olfactory and visual pathways. Kinetosis can be produced visually by observing the rise and fall of the horizon on a ship and by smells (oil, disinfectants, cooking) when combined with oscillatory movement. The phenomenon may be connected to conflicting impulses to the brain from the visual and labyrinthine sensors. These impulses are read in relation to a pattern of expected associations stored in the brain. The brain's failure to match perceived and received information results in conflict, dissonance and physiogical disturbance. It is generally accepted that motion sickness is a normal response to an abnormal environment.

One hypothesis postulates that the brain stem mechanisms of orientation and motion may perform an additional function, other than maintenance of body equilibrium, stability of head and body and gaze maintenance. This function detects and responds to certain poisons. With motion sickness, conflict in sensory inputs simulates poisoning in neuromechanisms (Treisman, 1977).

An alternative possibility is that there is a link between the perceptual motor adaptive processess and the onset of motion sickness.

An emetic chemo-receptor trigger zone (CTZ) in the area postrema of the medulla oblongata of the brain was thought to be implicated. When stimulated it would produce motion sickness. With certain forms of motion, a vomiting substance could be secreted into the cerebrospinal fluid in the emetic process (Borison, 1985). Ablation studies, however, suggest that the CTZ is not an essential component of the neural structures involved in motion sickness. Others believe that, an as yet unidentified neural element indispensable for the production of motion-induced vomiting, is located close to the area postrema.

Symptoms

Symptoms can present in varying degrees and may wax and wane. Vomiting initially eases the symptoms for a short period. Persistent vomiting over several days can result in dehydration and electrolyte inbalance, creating additional problems in those with diabetes meilitis, renal or hepatic problems. Recurrent vomiting can interfere with drug absorption and compliance in those on routine medication for chronic illness, or taking prophylactic antimalarials or oral contraceptives.

On long sea cruises, new cases of sea-sickness continue to appear after many hours if unaccustomed motion persists. Since stabilisers have been fitted on cruise vessels, the incidence has been reduced. However, in rough weather, passengers with the condition constitute the majority of the ship's doctor's patients (Oliver, 1977). Cruise shipping lines recognise the hazard to their passengers and provide antisickness pills free for prophylactic use. High flying modern aircraft can usually avoid turbulence but when it is encountered the unusual motion can quickly cause motion sickness. A sick bag is present in the pocket in front of every aircraft seat. Straight motorways with minor curves have reduced car sickness on British roads but winding lanes and highland roads still causes sickness in susceptible travellers. Metal strips fixed to the rear of cars are evidence that car sickness remains a common problem for passengers. In developing countries, roads are often little more than tracks. Car sickness caused by bouncing around in a poorly sprung vehicle on winding roads, affects many travellers. In the foothills and mountain areas, such as the Himalayas and the Andes, tourists are subjected to road travel over corkscrewing, climbing roads for many hours and often succumb to kinetosis. Cardinal signs and symptoms are:

- malaise
- cold sweats
- yawning
- abdominal discomfort
- pallor
- nausea
- vomiting
- cardiovascular symptoms
- frontal headache.

Cardiopulmonary disorder can be linked with:

- a racing pulse and tachycardia
- rapid, sometimes gasping, breathing
- changes in blood volume with pooling of blood in the lower parts of the body
- postural hypotension and syncope.

Psychological components present as varying degrees of :

- withdrawal
- apathy
- depression associated with functional incapacity.

Habituation

A feature of motion sickness is the individual's ability to become accustomed to types of motion. Most people get used to upsetting environmental stimuli over time. Conditioning is lost when exposure is discontinued and re-exposure to the disturbing motion is delayed for more than a few days. There is a conditioned susceptibility to motion sickness, and the threshold linking perceptual and motor adjustments of the sickness syndrome is subject to conditioning.

Habituation is also related to the pattern of motion. Habituation appears to involve a learning component, with the affected individual adapting postural control and locomotive function to the moving environment. In most cases of sea travel, passengers gain their 'sea legs' and adapt to the motion of the ship.

Studies of autonomic response in motion sickness simulation testing, show increases in pulse and ventilation rate and vasoconstriction. Some doctors believe that motion sickness can be categorised as a stress reaction, with people adapting to motion sickness as they do to other forms of stress (Cowing and Suter, 1986).

Precipitating factors

One cycle in 16 seconds is the frequency of up and down movement most likely to induce motion illness. Frequencies more than one cycle per second appear to produce little motion sickness in simulation studies. The sight or smell of food in preparation or on display, can encourage the development of the malaise. Kinetic sickness appears to be in part, an enduring psychological trait. Individuals who produce high scores in neuroticism, anxiety and introversion on rating scales, show a high correllation with susceptibility to travel sickness.

Air sickness has been considered by some to be a weakness associated with certain personality types eg. phobics, neurotics and the anxiety prone, who seem to be more susceptible to the effects of the psychological factors involved in air travel.

Motion sickness is likely to occur with any method of transport, if individuals are exposed to unaccustomed acceleration patterns. Its development can result from a broad range of physical stimuli, usually associated with changes in speed and direction. In cars and trains speed, sway and a tortuous route are likely triggers. Because an individual is seasick does not necessarily mean that he/she will also suffer air or car-sickness.

Predisposing factors

- ► fatigue
- ► alcohol consumption
- ► emotional state
- ► sleep deprivation
- ► some drugs can predispose to kinetic illness
- ► previous experience of travel sickness.

Other mammals, birds and even reptiles have been shown to suffer from motion sickness. Research has demonstrated that horses, pigs and cats suffer travel sickness.

Travellers in large ships can become ill on transfer to smaller boats and sailors can become sick when they transfer from a sailing vessel to an aircraft, and are exposed to air turbulence. The onset of kinetic sickness appears to depend on the frequency of the up and down movement specific to the mode of travel. There is no good predictive test of who is likely to suffer from motion sickness. Frequencies higher than one cycle per second of upward and downward movement rarely produce motion sickness. People transferring between transport modes with this oscillation are unlikely to see any difference in incidence of motion sickness. However, habituated passengers and sailors travelling in large ships often become sick when transferring to small boats with less stability than the parent ship. The closer the oscillation is to one cycle per second, the more likely it is that motion sickness will occur.

Preventive measures

- ▶ take up a horizontal position; lie flat if possible as this removes the vertical acceleration element of the motion
- ▶ keep the head fixed relative to the body, maintaining the eye gaze on the horizon
- ▶ if practical, avoid fixing the eyes on nearby moving objects
- ▶ reading should be avoided and closing the eyes helps.

In ships:

- ▶ occupy a mid-line position on board, close to the centre line of the ship on a mid-deck. This may help in stormy conditions
- ▶ midship cabins suffer less fore and aft oscillation
- ▶ book a cabin without portholes
- ▶ avoid alcohol and foods which have a high fat content
- ▶ clients who have Menieres disease are advised to avoid sea travel.

In a car:

- ▶ sit in the front seat with eyes fixed on the far horizon. Use a head rest to fix the head position
- ▶ use fresh air vents to avoid a hot stuffy atmosphere
- ▶ keep eyes fixed on the road ahead
- ▶ do not read
- ▶ changing the position of the driver's seat or changing drivers will usually abort impending car sickness.

In aircraft:

- ▶ the best place to sit is between the wings in the centre section
- ▶ sit as far from the kitchen as possible to avoid strong food smells.

Aircraft stability has greatly improved over the years. Motion and airsickness is less prevalent and usually occurs when flying low and in small aeroplanes.

Placebo effect

Simple remedies can be effective as there is a large placebo effect associated with travel-sickness therapy. Sea bands strapped to the wrists and exerting pressure over P6 acupuncture points are popular, so are metal strips placed on car bumpers. These remedies appear to prevent motion sickness for many people. Another popular remedy is to place a small cotton wool plug placed in one ear canal (always the opposite side from the person's right or left handedness) before travel. There is no scientific evidence on the efficacy of such remedies and the placebo effect may play a major role. Controlled therapy studies have shown that up to 55% of a group can benefit from appropriate drug therapy and 45% will benefit from placebo.

Altered attention and changes in concentration may also have beneficial psychological effects. Individuals committed to a specific cognitive task, such as navigation, driving or decision-making, are usually unaffected by motion sickness until their immediate attention and concentration is no longer required.

Drug therapy

Drug treatment can be a beneficial prophylactic for kinetoses. How they prevent travel-sickness is unknown although they may alter the susceptibility of the sensory organs involved in the disorder.

The two most common drug groups used, the phenothiazines and antihistamines, act centrally. The phenothiazines act on the chemoreceptor trigger zone (CTZ) and the vomiting centre and the antihistamines act on the CTZ and the vestibular apparatus. Both groups have anticholinergic side-effects which may be troublesome. Antihistamines are slower to take effect but have more persistent action. The benefits of both drug groups should be weighed against the potential side-effects to the patients if sea crossings or road journeys are short.

Drugs in general use are cinnarizine, cyclizine, dimenhydrinate, hyoscine, meclozine hydrochloride and promethazine.

A double-blind Norwegian study comparing 7 commonly used agents for prophylaxis of sea sickness in over 1700 volunteer tourists, showed little material difference in their efficacy. The scopalamine transdermal patch was marginally less effective, although its long action has benefits on sea voyages. Side-effects may persist for some hours after removal of the patch and they are unsuited for use in children.

There was no significant difference in the incidence and characteristics of adverse events related to drug medication, although the patch caused slightly more visual problems. The dryness of the mouth, which is associated with scopalamine, can be a major discomfort. However, its popularity with American tourists can be confirmed by the many drug patches in use on board cruise ships. It takes 6–8 hours for the drug to reach therapeutic level and it should be applied in advance of travel.

Due to the central action of effective travel-sickness drugs, clients are warned against drinking alcohol. Their use for car drivers or pilots is not recommended.

Of the drugs tested, cinnarizine, with domperidone, cyclizine, dimenhydrinate, ginger, and meclozine with caffeine may be recommended as prophylactics for seasickness. Cinnarazine in a dose of 150mg per day is currently favoured by many physicians.

People have their favourite remedies and with the very high placebo effect almost any anti-emetic is better than none.

Antihistamines are popular and can give protection for up to 24 hours. They cause sedation but this is often welcomed by travellers on long tedious journeys. They should not be used by decision-makers and drivers. Hyoscine has been many doctors' drug of choice for travel-sickness therapy for a long time.

Side-effects of drug therapy
dry mouth
dilated pupils
loss of visual acuity
a 'drugging' effect which causes lacklustre behaviour

Treatment of established motion sickness

Prophylaxis and avoidance behaviour is recommended. Once emesis is established, oral medication is of little value. An intramuscular injection of promethazine, 25–50mg, is the treatment of choice if sedation is not a problem. Kwell tablets dissolved in the mouth can be beneficial, and should be combined with trandermal patch application if exposure to the disturbing environmental motion is prolonged.

Although prophylactic drugs, favourite placebos, stabilised ships, high flying aeroplanes and better roads have reduced the incidence of travel asssociated sickness, it still afflicts many travellers. Drug treatment can offer some protection but has side-effects. The ideal travel-sickness remedy has not yet been found.

Useful drugs for travel sickness prophylaxis

Drug	Dose	Duration of effect
Dramamine	50mg dimenhydrinate 50mg caffeine	4 hours
Marzine	50mg cyclizine	4 + hours
Zintona	250mg ginger root	4 hours
Scopaderm	0.5mg scopolamine	72 hours
Stugeron	25mg cinannarazine	6 hours

Jet-lag

Crossing time zones in transmeridian travel causes jet-lag. Jet-lag is due to desynchronisation of internal body rhythms and persists until the traveller's body clock resynchronises. Alteration in the pattern of day and night cues causes external desynchronisation between circadian rhythms and the environment, ie. in Los Angeles it is late morning, but the body says its time to go to bed.

Modern aircraft circumnavigate the world and fly over northern and southern latitudes at almost the speed at which the earth rotates. Long transmeridian flights highlight the inability of human body systems to adjust rapidly to these changes. There is disparity beween the internal body clock and that of the external environment. Adjustment may take from a few days to a week or more. Correction rates are about 1.5 hours a day after flights to the west and 1 hour a day in flights to the east. Disruption is better tolerated after flights from east to west, rather than that from west to east. This phase of disruption is known as jet-lag.

Symptoms

- ▶ fatigue
- ▶ loss of vigour
- ▶ insomnia
- ▶ disturbed sleep
- ▶ irritability
- ▶ weakness
- ▶ sleep disruption is typical and often worst on the second night after arrival
- ▼ the severity of symptoms is determined by the number of time zones crossed and the direction of travel
- ▼ more symptoms are reported on return home than at a new destination (Petrie, 1989). This may relate to the amount of stimulation in the environment
- ▼ cumulative sleep loss is also a factor. Many transmeridian flights are overnight and result in conventional sleep loss

▼ clients who rise early and go to bed early appear to be more susceptible to jet-lag than those who are late risers and go to bed late

▼ older people are more susceptible and take longer to adjust to circadian changes

▼ westward flights are easier to adapt to, as it is easier to extend our day rather than to shorten it.

Treatment interventions

There are three possibilities:

► maximising alertness

► reducing sleep loss

► speeding up resynchronisation

Increase alertness with increased caffeine intake, ie. in tea, coffee and cola drinks. Also take physical exercise.

Improve sleep by avoiding caffeine at sleeping times. Sleep in a quiet dark room. Hypnotic medication may be taken for 2 or 3 nights after arrival and is most valuable on the second night. Hypnotics should not be taken for sleep disturbance after this initial period as there is no evidence of any effect on circadian rhythms in humans. Temazepam may help the client to sleep immediately after arrival but does nothing to re-establish circadian rythms (Donaldson and Kennoway, 1991).

Encouraging resynchronisation

Bright lights, exercise, diet and melatonin are possible countermeasures.

Bright light: in practical terms this means being in the open after arrival at the destination. Scheduled exposure to bright light (3000 lux) has been shown to speed up adjustment to transmeridian flights (Daan and Lewy, 1984). Bright light acts directly to influence melatonin. A few intrepid travellers can be seen on international airways wearing large brimmed hats carrying a gadget which switches bright lights into the wearer's eyes at programmed intervals. This may not combat jet lag but is a source of amusement to fellow passsengers using more mundane measures to avoid upset to circadian rhythms.

Exercise is effective in animals but has no proven value in humans.

Diet: there is no conclusive proof that diet has any effects, although high protein meals may have catecholamine activity and caffeine increases arousal.

Melatonin is a hormone secreted in the late evening which is suppressed by light. It has a key role in establishing circadian rhythms but melatonin therapy cannot eliminate jet-lag completely. Melatonin in 5–8mg doses, taken during the evening for 3 to 7 days after arrival at the destination appears to be effective in reducing jet-lag. Side-effects seem to be few but its use is still experimental. Currently the most promising therapy is the use of timed dose melatonin (Petrie and Dawson, 1994).

Although the effects of jet-lag are unavoidable, countermeasures can alleviate the symptoms. These are self-limiting and, for most travellers, acceptable.

Instruction leaflet for the traveller

If possible, choose direct and day time flights
Try to sleep on the aeroplane at the conventional sleeping time so that there is reduced sleep debt on arrival at the destination
Comply with the new environment time behaviour patterns on arrival
Avoid caffeine before the destination sleep time but it can be used for arousal if sleep threatens in the new day time
Avoid driving and business meetings immediately following arrival, after a long haul transmeridian flight
Avoid using sleeping pills to treat jet-lag
Try to organise global travel so that you fly east–west, rather than west–east

Dehydration

Dehydration is a medical threat to travellers in deserts and on mountains. Climbers on Kilimanjaro have to climb for two to three days with their own water supplies. The Alto Plano of the Peruvian and Bolivian Andes is especially arid and travel distances are determined by availability of water. In drought affected lands of East Africa and Asia, water is at a premium and may be infected. Backpackers and expeditioners often fail to carry sufficient fluid and, consequently, suffer dehydration on long journeys. High climbers lose fluid via the lungs, and need to drink enough water to allow for sustained effort and humidification of inspired air.

In desert conditions, dehydration and sunstroke are risks for expeditioners. Up to nine litres of fluid a day may be the minimum needed to maintain physical effort without fluid deprivation. Expeditioners should be encouraged to drink sufficient water to maintain a urinary frequency as close to normal as possible. Loss of salt can lead to electrolyte imbalance. One gramme of sodium chloride in one litre of water will help to avoid salt depletion (Melville, 1981).

Acclimatisation

The first few days in very hot zones are potentially the most dangerous. The traveller who is not yet acclimatised will secrete only half the volume of sweat as he/she will when acclimatised ten days later. Initial problems of body heat regulation carry a high risk of heat-stroke. Acclimatisation causes changes in the sweating mechanism and the blood circulating system to skin and limbs (Turner, 1971). Prior to acclimatisation, a man working hard outside, in extremes of heat (wet and dry), needs to drink nine litres of fluid a day (Steele and Franklin, 1980).

The most common forms of heat disorder

Heat syncope: a form of faint caused by sudden dilatation of the surface blood vessels, due to standing for a long time or working in extremes of heat.

Heat exhaustion: often caused by water or salt deficiency. It is commonly called heat stroke — a severe form of heat illness which can be fatal. As the body temperature rises rapidly, convulsions, kidney and liver damage can occur (Illingworth, 1984). With water deficiency the person begins to feel very hot and exhausted and with water depletion there is associated lethargy, lassitude and muscle cramps.

Heat pyrexia: is a serious condition usually affecting those not acclimatised. There is high fever, absence of sweating and unconsciousness soon occurs.

Prickly heat: is an annoying condition with itch and discomfort on parts of the body where air flow to the skin surface is restricted.

Prevention

These conditions can be avoided by drinking plenty of fluids, ensuring an adequate salt intake and by wearing light, cotton clothing.

High altitude hypoxia

Altitude effects are caused by the relative decrease in the partial pressure of oxygen which occurs with ascent from sea-level. With ascent, the atmospheric pressure falls and with it the partial pressure of oxygen. At 5500m both are at half normal.

High altitude illness syndromes, such as acute mountain sickness, high altitude pulmonary oedema (HAPE) and high altitude cerebral oedema (HACE) are primarily caused by this hypoxia. They can be life threatening and occur when climbers, who are not acclimatised to the resting altitude, make a high and rapid further ascent (see *Chapter 7*).

Categories of altitude

High altitude	2400m to 4300m (many ski resorts)
Very high altitude	4300 to 5500m (en route to Everest base camp)
Extreme altitude	5500m to 8848m (world's highest mountains)

Effects of hypoxia

Cardiac function is remarkably stable at altitude with the systemic arterioles dilating when exposed to low levels of oxygen. The main effect is on the pulmonary circulations with pulmonary arterioles constricting to hypoxia which can have catastrophic consequences. In hypoxia, arterial CO_2 rises and the hypoxic ventilatory response is triggered. People have periodic or Cheyne Stokes breathing patterns at altitude, particularly during sleep. At 400m, the normal sea level value for arterial oxygen saturation of 97%, will be reduced to 86% but will fall to 76% overnight.

Hypnotics have a depressant effect on the respiratory system and there is concern that they may cause desaturation of arterial oxygen. Hypnotic prescriptions for very high climbers, therefore, have not been recommended in the past. This may be true of the longer acting benzodiazepines and the barbiturates. However, a new study has shown that a small dose of temazepam improved the subjective quality of sleep at Everest base camp (5300m) and reduced changes in saturation without changing mean oxygen saturation (Dubowitz, 1998).

Acute mountain sickness (AMS) is the most common of the syndromes and, fortunately, the most benign.

Symptoms

• headache
• dizzyness
• breathlessness
• drowsiness
• anorexia
• nausea
• poor sleep

Skiers and climbers in the European Alps and the American Rocky Mountains may experience mild symptoms to which they will become acclimatised if staying and sleeping at lower altitudes. American ski resorts are becoming popular with British skiers and many fly into high ski areas. In one study of nearly 4000 people visiting ski resorts in Colorado between 2000 and 2880m altitude, 12% suffered from three or more symptoms of AMS (Houston, 1985). When skiers and trekkers fly in from lowlands to 2000m and ascend quickly to 4000m, almost half will suffer from AMS.

Very high climbers to the Himalayas and Andes are at considerable health risk from this disease as are those who fly in to high places from low level departure airports. Eighty-four percent of tour trekkers flying to the Hotel Everest (4205m) developed AMS. About 30,000 trekkers visit Nepal annually and many travel up to altitudes of 5500m — the height of Everest base camp.

Predictability

It is not possible to predict who will succumb to AMS. People under 20 years of age appear most likely to suffer, possibly because they over-exercise and do not pay attention to warning symptoms. Those who have had AMS before are likely to get it again, but there are no certain predictors of vulnerability. Going too far, too high and too fast are primary causes, but here is no relationship between susceptibility and physical fitness. It is more common in people who are cold and dehydrated.

High altitude pulmonary oedema (HAPE)

HAPE is often fatal and is a condition where there is a leak of high protein fluid into the lungs. Severe forms of AMS seem more common in men, with 49 men but only one woman being air rescued with HAPE, a potentially lethal complication of AMS, in a four year period in the Swiss Alps (Maggiorini, 1990). The approximate incidence of HAPE is 2% in those exposed to high altitude (Clarke, 1985). Risk factors include:

- ▶ the altitude gained — especially the sleeping altitude
- ▶ the rate of ascent
- ▶ heavy exertion
- ▶ hypnotic medication.

Symptoms

- ▶ dry cough
- ▶ decreased exercise performance
- ▶ breathless with exercise then tachycardia
- ▶ dyspnoea at rest

HAPE is characterised by breathlessness, cough and white frothy sputum which may become bloodstained.

Management

The illness requires early recognition, prompt descent and oxygen, and sublingual nifedipine. Immediate and rapid descent is required if the patient is to survive. If descent is impracticable, the patient should be placed in a Gamov bag if available. The fatality rate in high climbers was 4.3% in a study of British mountaineers, with 17% of those due to HAPE. The condition has contributed to many of the recorded fatal trauma deaths on high mountains (Pollard, 1988).

High altitude cerebral oedema (HACE)

This is the presence of progressive neurological deterioration in someone with AMS or HAPE.

Symptoms

▶ ataxia and stupor with rapid progression to coma.

HACE is characterised by severe headaches, irrational behaviour, errors of judgement, hallucinations and ataxia which can rapidly progress to unconsciousness. The victim suffers the symptoms of raised intracranial pressure. Immediate and rapid descent is mandatory if the individual is to survive both these conditions.

Management

Prompt descent, oxygen and steroids. If descent is difficult then a Gamov bag should be used.

Prophylaxis and treatment

The carbonic anhydrase inhibitor, acetazolamide, makes the cerebrospinal fluid more acidic and this, as a consequence, drives the medullary respiratory centre and prevents deoxygenation. Prophylaxis for AMS may be achieved by a dose of 125mg to 250mg per day, started 24 hours before climbing above 3000m (Green *et al*, 1980; McIntosh and Prescott, 1986).

A reasonable climbing programme below 4300m is to climb at a rate of up to 300m daily. Above this level this should be 150 to 300m per day with every third day a rest day. This may be a counsel of perfection but allows acclimatisation.

Acetazolamide may also be used in the treatment of AMS and periodic breathing. A usual side-effect of this drug is peripheral paraesthesia with annoying but tolerable electric shock tinglings in the arms and legs.

AMS can be avoided by allowing acclimatisation to occur during a slow graded ascent to higher altitude and sleeping as low as possible at night. Return to a low level altitude will normally reverse milder forms of AMS.

People at special risk

Risks are higher in people with cardiopulmonary disease. If they suffer from high blood pressure, with possible occlusive arterial disease, they should seek medical advice, or attend a travel health clinic for counselling, before venturing above 4000m on a sports trip. Diabetes mellitis, controlled epilepsy, hypertension and asthma are not in themselves contraindications to travelling to high altitude. However, if people are sports enthusiasts, the disorders may be compounded by the effects of exercise and high altitude.

High altitude travel presents special health risks which should be considered by the health professional in the travel clinic and the nurse and doctor in the surgery. People going to a high altitude destination should be counselled on the health problems which might present and and advised on how to avoid and prevent them.

Information leaflet

• be aware of the health risks associated with high altitude (over 3000m)
• below 4300m climb at a rate of no more than 400m daily
• above 4300m climb at 150–300m daily
• consider taking acetazolamide to help avoid acute mountain sickness if climbing above 3000m
• do not go too far, too high and too fast at altitude
• endeavour to sleep low at night and climb high by day
• if symptoms of AMS appear and the headache does not resolve with paracetamol, descend
• avoid long-acting sleeping pills at high altitude
• take plenty of fluid daily

Cabin hypoxia

Hypoxia can occur in the cabin of high flying aircraft. Air pressures are usually artificially mantained at a level higher than sea level, about 200–300m. This may mean that people with respiratory and cardiac problems suffer hypoxia.

References

Borison L (1985) Motion sickness. *Aviat Space Environ Med* **56**: 66–8

Clarke C (1985) Diseases of high altitude.*Update* 862–8

Cowing S, Suter S (1986) Motion sickness. *Psychophysiol* **23**: 542–51

Daan S, Lewy A (1984) Scheduled exposure to daylight. *Psychpharmacol Bull* **15**: 566–8

Donaldson E, Kennoway D (1991) Effects of temazepam on sleep melatonin and cortisol excretion after transmeridian travel. *Aviat. Space Environ Med* **62**: 654–60

Dubowitz G (1998) Effect of temazepam on oxygen saturation and sleep at high altitude. *Br Med J* **316**: 587–9

Green M, Kerr A, McIntosh IB (1981) *Br Med J* **283**: 811–13

Guyton A (1976) *Textbook of Medical Physiology*, 4th edn. WB Saunders, Philadelphia

Houston CS (1985) Incidence of AMS. *Am Alpine J* **27**: 161–2

Illingworth R (1984) *Expedition Medicine: A planning guide*. Blackwell Scientific Press, Oxford

Maggiorini M, Buhler B, Walter M *et al* (1990) Prevalence of acute mountain sickness in the Swiss Alps. *Br Med J* **301**: 853–5

McIntosh IB, Prescott R (1986) Acetazolamide in the prophylaxis of acute mountain sickness. *J Int Med Res* **14**: 285–7

Melville K (1981) *Stay Alive in the Desert*. Lascelles, London

Oliver PO (1977) Health problems of passengers at sea. *Practitioner* **219**: 210–14

Oosterveld WA (1997) *Motion Sickness: Textbook of Travel Medicine and Health*. BC Decker, Hamilton

Petrie K, Conaglen J, Thompson L (1989) Effect of melatonin on jet-lag after long haul flights. *Br Med J* **298**: 705–7

Petrie K Dawson AG (1994) Recent developments in the treatment of jet-lag. *J Trav Med* **2**: 79–83

Pollard A, Clarke C (1988) Deaths during mountaineering at extreme altitude. *Lancet* : 1277

Steele P, Franklin J (1980) Getting it together. In: Cranfield I, ed. *The Independent Traveller's Handbook*. Heineman, London

Treisman M (1977) Motion sickness: an evolutionary hypothesis. *Science* **197**: 493–5

Turner A (1971) *The Travellers Health Guide*. Stacie, London

Velimirovic B (1990) Health hazards of sea tourism. *Trav Med Int* **8**: 69–74

Appendix I

Dangers from the sun while abroad

Over exposure to the sun can not only cause severe sunburn but also heat stroke, dehydration and cancer of the skin.

- ► The closer to the equator the holiday destination, the greater are the effects of the sun's rays. For example, in southern Spain the sun's rays are twice as harmful as in the UK

- ► Adverse effects from the sun are greatest, between 10am and 3pm

- ► Graded exposure for short intervals of under half an hour protects against the adverse effects of the sun

- ► High reflection on beaches, by the water increases the burning effects of the sun. Its rays can pass through lightly woven materials such as thin shirts and blouses. Adequate protection can only be obtained from sun screen lotions and creams with protection factors above 10. These should be applied frequently to the children's skin and to that of fair-skinned adults

- ► Skin cancer is a serious risk for fair skinned, blued-eyed, red and fair haired people who freckle. The effects of the rays build up with continued exposure over a number of years. The risk is only minimised by avoiding direct exposure to sunlight from 10am to 3pm and by with frequent applications of high factor protective sun lotions and creams. Too much sun can kill.

- ► Cloud cover may be misleading. The heat of the sun is reduced and the danger is less obvious. People stay out in shaded sunlight for longer and, as ultra violet light pass through light cloud cover, the sun's rays can still cause sunburn.

- ► Ultra violet light reflection from the surface of water is also a danger. Sand reflects a quarter of light rays and thre quarters of the sun's rays will be transmitted through water, affecting swimmers even below the surface.

► The higher the sun is above the horizon, the shorter is the parth of the rays and the greater the risk of sunburn.

Appendix II

Vaccinations and malaria prevention

People return from holiday and frequently develop malaria, which can be fatal. Increased resistance to drug therapy means that many are inadequately protected.

Over much of Asia, India, Africa and South America, there is a high risk of malaria infection. Travellers to these areas should start appropriate medication one week prior to departure on holiday and continue for six weeks after their return.

Active prevention

Mosqitoes are the source of malaria infection and it cannot be assumed that taking drugs is sufficient to protect the individual.

- ▶ Long trousers, long-sleeved blouses and shirts should be worn for protection against insect bites. Exposed areas of the face, hands and neck should be protected with preparations, such as DEET or Jungle Formula, which can be purchased from the chemist

- ▶ Hotel rooms should be sprayed with appropriate anti-mosquito repellents or a pyrrethrum coil should be lit to deter the insects

- ▶ Even transient visits, as short as an hour or two to infected areas, can result in infection. People in transit stops on air journeys have been infected at airports.

Vaccination against other diseases

Cholera and typhoid, hepatitis and AIDS are common in many parts of the world. All travellers who live in the UK should ensure that they have been vaccinated against poliomyelitis and tetanus. If there is a risk of cholera, typhoid, yellow fever or hepatitis, they should also arrange for appropriate vaccination.

Random sexual encounters is Asia and Africa have a high risk of infection with HIV and the later development of AIDS. The use of condoms decreases the risk but does not wholly protect. In the absence of a cure, abstinence is the only certain means of protection.

Dental needles, chiropody instruments and injections can transmit disease in parts of Asia and Africa, and treatment should be avoided if at all possible when abroad.

Appendix III

Contaminated water spreads disease when abroad

Contaminated water is a frequent cause of diarrhoea in travellers. Outside western Europe and North America, the water is nearly always suspect. It may also be contaminated along the shores of the Mediterranean.

When travelling it is better to assume that water supplies harbour disease. Hotel tap water should be sterilised with Puritabs and in the tropics, Asia and Africa, sterilised water should even be used for cleaning teeth.

Water can be sterilised by adding Puritabs (purchased from any chemist) and it will be ready for consumption with half an hour of treatment. The iodine taste can be disguised by adding orange powder.

Water can also be sterilised by boiling and by using a traveller's kettle or electric coil.

Ice for drinks is a frequent source of contamination and the addition of ice cubes to drinks should be avoided. Ideally, only commercially bottled water should be drunk or carbonated water. In some countries, such as India and China, even the commercial supplies may be contaminated.

Diarrhoea and vomiting requires treatment by fluid replacement. This means copious input in small amounts.

If diarrhoea and vomiting occur, drink flat coke or carbonated drinks. The necks of bottles or the tops of tins of commercial drinks also carry disease and they should be cleaned with wet, medicated wipes before drinking directly from them.

It is wise to carry a packet of drinking straws on global journeys. If used to sip drinks, they reduce the risk of infection from contaminated bottle tops or cups.

Fruit and vegetables are often washed in contaminated water and salads should be avoided if the water source is suspect.

Appendix IV

Infected food can cause disease

▶ Diarrhoeal illness is very common in travellers and can spoil the holiday

▶ Diarrhoeal illness is avoidable with precautions

▶ Most travellers' diarrhoea is caused by swallowing contaminated food and drink

▶ Diarrhoeal illness is usually self-limiting and wil get better after one to three days with no treatment other than replacement of body losses

Hints on safe eating and and drinking abroad

Food choice:

▶ Choose food that is freshly cooked.

▶ Freshly boiled food is always safe, eg. rice.

▶ Peel all fruit and vegetables before eating.

▶ Eat food from sealed packs or cans.

▶ Do not eat: salads, shellfish, unpeeled fruit or vegetables, ice-cream and ices.

▶ Sauces and relishes left out on the table or food on which insects have settled will be infected.

▶ Remember, contaminated plates and cutlery not washed with detergent or rinsed in clean water and protected from flies, can cause infection.

▶ Hands and fingers should be washed at every opportunity, preferably in water with added disinfectant.

▶ Only eat food that you have handled if your hands are scrupulously clean.

Drinking water

Outside western Europe and North America, drinking water is nearly always suspect and should be boiled before use or sterilised with 'Puritabs'.

Ice is often frozen, contaminated water. Ice cubes and iced drinks spread disease.

If in doubt, if food is not cooked, boiled or peeled, avoid it.

Sources of information

The complexity of modern travel with ever-changing recommendations and legal requirements for entry into different countries means that general practitioners running travel clinics need access to authoritative and up-to-date information.

The Scottish Centre for Infection and Environmental Health (SCIHE) offers its own computerised database free to GPs throughout Scotland, with a small fee for other Gps in the UK who contact them by telephone. GPs with suitable computer equipment can gain direct access to this database via TRAVAX. The TRAVAX system gives recommendations for immunisations on malaria prophylaxis and also warns of outbreaks of infectious disease throughout the world.

Information sources

Scottish Centre for Infection and Environmental Health (SCIEH)
Clifton House
Clifton Place
Glasgow, G3 7LN

Dept of Health
Alexander Fleming House
Elephant and Castle
London, SE1 6BY
Tel: 0171 972 2000

Dept of Communicable and Tropical Diseases
East Birmingham Hospital
Bordesley Green Road
Birmingham, B9 5ST
Tel: 0121 766 6611

Dept of Infectious Diseases
Monsall Hospital
Manchester, M10 8WR
Tel: 0161 205 2393

Hospital for Tropical Diseases
4 St Pancras Way
London, NW1 0PE
Tel: 0171 387 4411

Holiday Care Service
2 Old Bank Chambers, Station Rd
Harley, Surrey
Tel: 01293 774535

Liverpool School of Tropical Medicine
Pembroke Place
Liverpool, L3 5QA
Tel: 0151 708 9393

RADAR (Royal Association for Disability and Rehabilitation)
25 Mortimer Street
London, W1N 8AB
Tel: 0171 637 5400

Ross Institute of Tropical Hygiene
London School of Hygiene and Tropical Medicine, Keppel Street
London, WC1E 7HT
Tel: 0171 636 8636

British Diabetic Association
10 Queen Anne Street
London, W1M 0BD
Tel: 0171 323 1531

Merieux Vaccination Information Service
Merieux UK
Clivemont House, Clivemont Road
Maidenhead, Berkshire, F16 7BU
Tel: 01628 786291

London School of Hygiene and Tropical Medicine
Malaria Reference Laboratory
(Malaria only)
T3l: 0171 636 7921

Department of Health
International Relations Division
Tel 0171 407 5522, Ext. 6711

British Heart Foundation
14 Fitzharding Street
London, W1H 4DH

Sterile Medical Equipment Pack
(Suitable for single adult)
Available from MASTA Ltd
Keppel Street, London, WC1E 7HT
Tel 0171 631 4408

Travel AIDS Kit
Available from Philip Harris Medical Ltd
Hazelwell Lane, Stirchley
Birmingham, B30 2PA

Index

cyano bacteria 59
cyanobacteria 77
cyclizine 127
D
deaf 36-37
death 17
death rate 29
decompression sickness 61, 71
deep venous thrombosis 28
dehydration 52, 62, 71, 76-77, 131
desensitisation 114
desynchronisation 129
desynchronisation of circadian rhythm 103
diabetes 11, 80
diabetes mellitus 45, 122, 137
diarrhoea 62
dimenhydrinate127
disease 70
    cardiac 28
    respiratory 28
disturbance to circadian rhythm 119
diving injuries 58
douching
    rectal64
    vaginal 64
drowning 46, 50, 58, 73
drug absorption 122
drug interaction 81
drug misuse 21
drug therapy 127
drugs 17-18, 111
drugs for travel sickness prophylaxis 128
dysentery 11
E
'en route' psychological trauma 98
ear infections 59
elderly 110
elderly travellers 32
enclosed spaces 108
endemicity 87, 94
epilepsy 45, 137
evacuation 78
exposure 71
extreme cold 42
extremes of temperature 70
eye injury 48

F
facial structure
    haemorrhages 66
falling 108
falls 29, 34, 50
fear of heights 108
fears 25, 98, 104, 108
    air travel 100
    flying 98
fever 62
fire 32, 34
first aid facilities 34
first-aid kit 74, 80
flight delays 111
flooding 114
fluid loss 52
flying anxieties 19
food allergy 30
food poisoning 11
fracture
    to hips 33
    to spine 33
fractures 29, 34, 50, 63
frostbite 42, 71
frost-nip 42
G
galley scalds 77
gastroenteritis 74, 77
gastrointestinal 79
gravel burns 63
greenstick fracture 49
group psychology 83
guinea worm 60, 77
H
habituation 123
HACE
    See Also high altitude cerebral oedema
haemoconcentration 52
haemorrhages of the eye 66
haemotoma 77
HAPE 45, 135
    See Also high altitude pulmonary oedema
HBV 86
head injuries 47, 50
health professional, role of 105
health risks 70
health status 80